INTRODUCTION

Your fifth chakra is best introduced with a Hindu story.

According to Indian mythology, the battle between good and evil has always taken place between *devas* (gods) and *rakshasas* (demons). During one such skirmish, Vishnu, the male god devoted to preservation, attempted to resolve the fight by churning the ocean, which represents the world and the mind. What emerged from the swirling waters was the nectar of immortality. This nectar gave life but was also a poison.

The devas received the nectar, but no one wanted the harmful poison. So another god stepped up.

Shiva, representing the power of destruction, drank the nectar. By doing so, he neutralized the danger. Most of the venom lodged in his throat. While he rendered the poison harmless, his neck turned blue. The remainder of the venom, which Shiva shared with the world, now had the ability to transmute any contaminants in the body and activate the higher powers, leading to enlightenment.

Because of Shiva's selfless gift, we can activate our own abilities through this same throat-based energy center, named *vishuddha* in Hinduism. The term means "purification" in Sanskrit, an ancient and symbolic language. Today, we most often call this center the fifth chakra (or throat chakra) and love interacting with it for the amazing gifts it promises.

We all want to reach for our highest potential while simultaneously defusing the toxic elements of life. Because of the capabilities this chakra brings to this aspiration, I have personally labeled it the "pure nectar" chakra. As one of many subtle energy centers that manage all areas of your life, its duties can be most easily summarized in a single word: communication.

Through this blue-colored energy center, we learn to be more discriminating, creative, and self-expressive. As we heal the blocks in this energy center, we transmute negative experiences into wisdom. Sound becomes a vehicle for higher truths, and we find ourselves able to hear and listen from our most genuine nature, which is spiritual. As we purify our communication, we purify ourselves.

It is my joy to be your main guide to your fifth/throat chakra, the topic of this book and the fifth in an eight-book series called Llewellyn's Chakra Essentials.

In the same way we ascend a ladder, we began our chakra journey at rung one, initiating our climb with a book encompassing the first chakra, the *muladhara*/root chakra. The second book climbed from the root to the second chakra, *svadhisthana*, found in the abdomen.

Upward we climbed to rung three, next introducing the *manipura*/solar plexus chakra. The fourth book in the series featured *anahata*, the heart chakra, the source of love. Now you have landed on rung five, an in-depth embrace of your fifth chakra, located in the throat.

Each book after this one will constitute yet another stairstep in the ascension toward the heavens, culminating in the eighth book, which features five out-of-body extraordinary chakras; I'll share a bit more about those special chakras later. Just because this is a series, however, doesn't mean you need to read and enjoy these books in any special order. Like the stars in the sky, each occupies its own special zone in the vast universe. Make transformative changes in one chakra, and gains show up in the others. That's because they are all linked through the physical and subtle self.

In the physical realm, every living being is equipped with seven in-body chakras that are based in the spine. These energy bodies numerically march upward from the base (first chakra) to the top of the head (seventh chakra). Given this ordering, you can perceive why I used a ladder analogy to introduce you to the first seven books in our series; the in-body chakras are literally stacked atop one another.

Each of these seven chakras is also rooted in an endo-crine gland and manages distinct bodily processes. The same is true of the out-of-body chakras as the body proper is the interconnection between all subtle centers. Spe-cifically, within your pure nectar chakra lie most of your throat-based bodily parts, including your parathyroid, jaw, mouth, neck, hearing apparatus, and thyroid, the major hormone gland of this energy center. The functions related to these and other body parts within this area are governed by your fifth chakra.

Your chakras are tasked with running more than physical concerns. Each is also in charge of aspects of your psycho-logical and intuitive activities.

Psychologically, your fifth chakra represents the emo-tional factors related to listening, interpreting, articulating, and withholding. Balance in this chakra results when you can pivot gracefully between the drives for reflection versus expression and quietude versus loudness.

The spiritual capacity of this chakra includes the apti-tude for gathering and deciphering everyday as well as psy-chic guidance. That's right: this chakra receives messages from otherworldly realms. As such, it plays a vital role in the development of enlightenment, which partially depends on our ability to receive advice from on high. Once we develop the skill of separating lies from truths and wasteful information from beneficial data, this chakra is ready to receive the golden nectar of enlightenment that I mentioned at the beginning of this introduction. You'll learn much more about both the physical and metaphysical origins of that nectar in the first part of this book.

For background, we must ask the ancient Hindus to take a bow for providing the modern world with the term *chakra*. The source language of the Indus Valley was Sanskrit, and the earliest of these people employed the word *chakra* to mean "spinning wheel of light." However, many cultures acknowledge the existence of these energy centers. Other groups that do include the ancient and current Inca, Cherokee, Hopi, Hebrew, Mayan, Aztec, Berber, and African Kemetic groups. No matter your own ethnic background, chances are that the spiritual medicine of your lineage has professed the existence of nonapparent energy bodies.

Although they are described as spheres of light, chakras are also made of sound; thus, they mirror the same substances that formulate all living beings. Absolutely everything is composed of oscillating energetic fields of light and sound, or energy.

Energy is information that moves. Spiritual masters across time, as well as present-day scientists, know the truth that energy composes everything. The caveat is that there are two types of energy: physical and subtle.

Physical energy creates measurable reality. Biologically, these tangible energies are run by physical organs, channels, and fields. However, more than 99.999 percent of any object, including your body, is made of subtle energy.[1] Achieving the good life certainly requires knowledge of your physical structures and subcomponents, but even these are mainly managed by subtle energies and their related structures.

Just as your physical energies are organized by organs, channels, and fields, so are your subtle energies. Altogether, these three subtle structures add up to your subtle energy anatomy, which is also called the subtle body.

Although this entire book is about your fifth chakra, and the series is devoted to the twelve chakras, I want to apprise you of two other subtle energy structures. This is because they overlap with your chakras and prove the assertion I made earlier in this introduction that all your chakras are interconnected, as are all your subtle energy systems. This also means they continually impact one another.

---

1   Ali Sundermier, "99.9999999% of Your Body Is Empty Space," Sciencealert, September 23, 2016, https://www.sciencealert .com/99-9999999-of-your-body-is-empty-space.

As far as subtle channels go, there are two main types: meridians and nadis.

Meridians are like riverways that pass through your connective tissue. These carry both physical and subtle energies throughout your body. They are mainly explained in traditional Chinese medicine (TCM), although worldwide, other subtle medicine systems also feature these subtle channels. The other journey-way, the *nadis,* are a Hindu construct. They are tantamount to your nerves. Both your nadis and meridians exchange energy with your seven in-body chakras.

Every chakra also creates its own field of subtle energy, called an *auric field* or *auric layer.* These individual emanations surround your body, one atop the other. Altogether, the entire sphere formulates the *auric field.* Every single layer serves a protective function. Based on the programming inside its associated chakra, it determines which energies can enter or exit that chakra. As you might guess, we'll be exploring your fifth auric field in this book, as it's an extension of your fifth chakra.

We have now arrived at the discussion I teased a bit earlier. There is an eighth book in this series that features five chakras beyond the seven in-body ones. Yes, I teach a twelve-chakra and twelve–auric field system. One of the reasons I have included these five out-of-body chakras in my thirty-plus books is that I perceived them as a child.

As a kid, I could see colorful balls and streams of light surrounding people and animals, even emanating from plants and trees. I didn't know it at the time, but I realized later that I was able to perceive subtle energy.

My parents were quite Christian, the type that didn't go in for anything as amorphous as "energy." Chakras weren't covered in Sunday school. But that blip in my spiritual education didn't keep me from noticing those beautiful hues of rainbow lights or from noticing that there were twelve specific spheres: seven expressing from individuals' spines and five floating around their bodies, always in the same places. Their appearance assisted me in making everyday decisions.

For instance, when my mom's bright red first chakra glowed with a ferocious flame, I knew I was going to get in trouble and I would run or hide. If my dad's usually cheery second chakra shifted from a clear orange to a muddy brown, I knew he would drink a lot that night.

At about age twenty, I started traveling the world to learn about these energies from healers, shamans, intuitives, and gurus in places including Japan, Peru, Venezuela, Morocco, Costa Rica, and Belize. My teachers knew about chakra-like energies as well as other subtle energy structures. Over the years, I added scientific studies to my bailiwick while continuing to invest in additional cross-cultural explorations. I wasn't really surprised to discover that there is nothing imperative about working with only seven chakras, the model used in the West since the early 1900s. The truth is that chakra-based and other spiritual medicine systems from around the world have depicted anywhere from three to dozens of chakras.

My first book featured my twelve-chakra system. Published through Llewellyn decades ago, my model has since become internationally renowned. You'll love learning about five additional out-of-body chakras in the eighth book in this series.

Back to the present.

There are two parts to this book. I am the sole author of part 1, which consists of three chapters that feature the fundamentals about your throat chakra. Most of the data is sourced from the classical Hindu bed of knowledge, though applicable modern concepts are interspersed. Throughout part 1 are practices aimed at helping you customize the material to your own life.

In the first chapter, I'll cover fifth chakra basics. Included are topics such as the throat chakra's main purpose and location, historical names, color, and sound. I also share information about associated elements, breaths, lotus petals, and the affiliated god and goddess, as well as knowledge about the nadis and that amazing golden nectar.

In chapter 2 I'll dive into the physicality of your fifth chakra. Like all in-body chakras, your pure nectar center is anchored within its own region of your spine. Because it is also linked to an endocrine gland and other bodily regions, subtle and physical damage to this area can result in any number of disease processes, which I'll describe in some detail. In chapter 3 I'll delve into the psychological and spiritual functions of this brilliant blue energy body.

Then onward we move into part 2, the focus of which is how to create your optimum life by mining and applying the energies of your fifth chakra.

Part 2 begins with an informative introduction to intention, your foremost healing and manifesting tool for the chapters that follow. Also provided is a guided meditation to assist you with tapping into your fifth chakra. Then comes the fun part: you'll meet new friends.

Each chapter in part 2 is authored by an energy expert. You'll kick off with an exploration of your fifth chakra spiritual allies before stretching into fifth chakra yoga poses. On and on you'll skip, hop, and deep dive, acquiring an intensely practical tool kit of fifth chakra practices. These tools will include the use of guided meditation, vibrational remedies, stones, sounds, shapes, colors, and even recipes.

In the end, you will avail yourself of what the Hindus saw as the nectar of the gods: the golden drops of purity that can enable communication as well as a lovely sense of self-knowledge.

PART 1

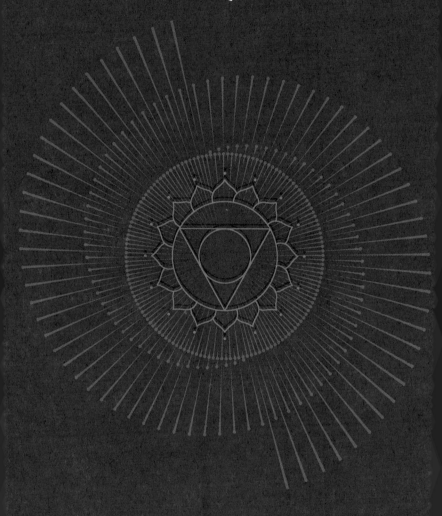

ESTABLISHING THE FOUNDATION
OF YOUR FIFTH CHAKRA KNOWLEDGE

• • • • • •

Place your tongue on the roof of your mouth, called the palate. For one round of breath, inhale and exhale deeply through your nose. On the next round, breathe in and out through your mouth. Then return your tongue softly to its usual resting position.

Now breathe naturally while visualizing shades of blue you find appealing: bright, shiny, soft, medium, sky, azure, indigo, cobalt, turquoise, sea . . . it's your choice. Mix and match blues as you desire.

Then imagine these streams of color rolling around in your mouth, cleansing and cleaning, before radiating outward to fill in empty spots and erase congestion in your throat and neck area. Remain in this free flow of blue until this area is completely relaxed.

When you're ready, take a couple of additional deep breaths and return to your everyday awareness. Be assured that these blue beams will continue creating ease and calm for as long as necessary.

You have just interacted with your fifth chakra.

In part 1, which lies ahead, you'll enjoy learning all about this blue chakra. I'll mainly present the essential fundamentals from Hindu culture, although I'll also sprinkle in enough contemporary knowledge and practices to thoroughly acquaint you with its potent powers.

In the first chapter, I'll lay out details about this chakra's main characteristics. Included will be subjects ranging from its location and related elements to its associated gods and goddesses. In chapter 2 I'll outline the physical functions of your pure nectar center before shifting into chapter 3, which will explore this chakra's psychological and spiritual qualities. My hope is that this information will float into your mind like drops of gentle rain, leaving you bathed in the poetry of your own throat chakra.

1

FUNDAMENTALS

Think about how much time you spend in reflection or expression. Humans are communicative creatures; it seems we are always talking, singing, humming, writing, learning, or philosophizing. Even if we're quiet, we're at least ruminating. Of course, silence qualifies as its own form of articulation.

Your fifth chakra, that all-essential blue energy center anchored in your throat, is your major gateway of communication. Situated between your head and your body proper, it interconnects your brain and your active self. It is via this energy center that you assess your personal truths and decide whether to convey them or not—whether to act upon them or do nothing at all. One reason it's so beneficial to understand all facets of your fifth chakra is that it will help you make more conscious decisions about every form of communication, which is key to developing healthy exchanges in all areas of life.

In this chapter, I'll first introduce you to Manisha, a real person (name changed) whose entire life improved once she cleaned up the dysfunctional beliefs within her fifth chakra and began interacting through it with more assurance. I'll then treat you to several mini sections that feature the most vital aspects of standard fifth chakra teachings. Much of this data is culled from Hindu tradition, which means it is thousands of years old. Some is contemporary, including modern spiritual and scientific knowledge. The criterion I've used to determine what to include here can be summed up simply: It is beneficial.

The information about your fifth chakra that might best benefit you will be outlined, discussed, illuminated, and then packaged into a couple of practices so you can immediately integrate this knowledge into your everyday life. My hope is that the pure nectar of your own golden wisdom will be called forth to empower all your communications as well as your moments of silence.

THE ESSENCE OF YOUR FIFTH CHAKRA

Manisha found her way to my office through her general practitioner. He was a functional medical doctor, which means he assessed challenges through both allopathic and holistic lenses. He put Manisha on thyroid medication but also suggested she work with me as well as a therapist.

Why? He believed that her Hashimoto's disease was caused by deep energetic and emotional issues he wasn't qualified to address.

There are many diseases of the thyroid, the main endocrine gland associated with the throat chakra. Several of these fit into the category of autoimmune disorders, which occur when the body's immune system erroneously attacks healthy cells. With Hashimoto's disease, the immune system creates antibodies that treat the thyroid cells as microbes or foreign agents. Symptoms are varied, from fatigue to cold sensitivity. A single mother, Manisha was struggling to keep up with her two teenagers and hold down a full-time job while dragging herself through her days.

Your fifth chakra might be the center of communication, but it also manages much of your physical health. For example, the thyroid produces hormones that govern everything from energy levels to the ability to sleep. In the case of Hashimoto's disease, which results in hypothyroidism, or the production of too few thyroid hormones, challenges often cause depressed moods, an erratic heartbeat, sexual dysfunction, drowsiness, and a generally lackluster approach to life.

As an energy healer, I employ my intuition to help clients determine the causal factors underlying their symptoms.

The range of potential causes is vast, as they can include issues from past and in-between lives, ancestral inheritances, family-of-origin dysfunctions, this-life events, and so much more. Core problems can reduce to physical, psychological, or spiritual considerations or a complicated array of these influences.

When interacting with a client, I often first figure out which chakra to focus on as a starting point. In Manisha's case, it was obvious I should first peruse her fifth chakra; after all, the thyroid is a critical component of this energy center.

I intuitively peered into Manisha's pure nectar chakra and saw her holding her hands over her ears while her parents screamed at each other. That picture was worth a thousand words.

After I shared this image aloud, Manisha started crying. Indeed, she agreed, her parents had argued during her entire childhood. If she tried to interrupt them or share her feelings about their fights, then they would yell at her. Sometimes they would lock her in her room. Little wonder that Manisha learned to lock away her thoughts and needs inside the closet of her fifth chakra. As a result, her thyroid responded by functioning as poorly as her communication abilities. Even as an adult, when she was being neglected or mistreated, she wouldn't speak up. In fact, she hadn't asked for a raise at work in years despite carrying a hefty amount of the responsibility in her department. Neither did she request that her children perform any chores, which left her to manage the entire household by herself.

Manisha started keeping a journal recording all the thoughts and emotions she had wanted to voice as a child and shared it with me and her therapist. Eventually she realized that she was running her life based on ideas like "Expression is dangerous" and "No one cares what I desire or feel." As she said to me after a few weeks of sessions, "My thyroid is as shut down as I am."

While working through her past, Manisha became brave enough to start sharing her truths in her everyday life. To boost her confidence, she used several of the subtle energy tools you'll learn in part 2; for instance, she employed affirmations when feeling down and vibrational remedies to transform her inner thoughts. She also called upon spirit allies for advice. Once, a being she called her angel told her exactly how to talk to a friend who was taking advantage of her.

After a few months, Manisha took on her boss by asking for a promotion. When she was turned down, she resigned and was immediately snapped up by another company, with a huge jump in pay.

I wasn't surprised that Manisha's fifth chakra energetic work improved her energy levels and hormone counts. As her need for prescription medication waned, her physician weaned her down to a nominal amount. The last time I saw Manisha, she was glowing. She was taking her kids on a much-needed vacation. They had fulfilled enough household duties to earn a skiing trip, and Manisha could hardly wait to get on the slopes.

Whenever we're able to work energetically, we're bound to experience an upswing in all life areas. By finessing your fifth chakra, you can potentially improve anything from hormone function to self-confidence, relationships to self-esteem. To make sure the evidence of this shows up in your everyday life, pay special attention to the following sets of data. By learning about your fifth chakra, you are essentially gaining an education about yourself.

OVERARCHING PURPOSE

Your fifth chakra is the seat of communication and expression, governing the ability to embrace and present truth.

IT'S ALL IN THE NAME: TERMS FOR THE FIFTH CHAKRA

The Sanskrit word for this chakra, *vishuddha*, means "purification." Tantric names include *akasha* and *kantha*. Akasha is also the name of the gross element associated with this chakra; you'll learn more about it in the section devoted to that topic later in this chapter.

LOCATION OF THE FIFTH CHAKRA

The fifth chakra is aligned with the base of the throat and is mainly associated with the cervical plexus, a collection of nerves physically located at the back of the neck and the base of the head, and secondarily with the pharyngeal plexus, which is associated with the throat.

COLOR OF THE FIFTH CHAKRA

A chakra runs on a unique set of frequencies. In turn, frequencies are organized as bandwidths that are describable as specific ranges of colors and sounds. I'll cover the sound of your pure nectar chakra in the next section.

The coloration of your fifth chakra relates to the range of frequencies we call blue. Blue is a spectrum that is measurable by scientists, who describe it as operating on a wavelength of about 450 to 495 nanometers in the visible light spectrum. For perspective, blues are the shortest rays of light that can be seen by the human eye. Blue also holds a lot of energy; in fact, it carries more punch than colors like green and red. It is also one of three primary colors, meaning it isn't produced by combining other colors.

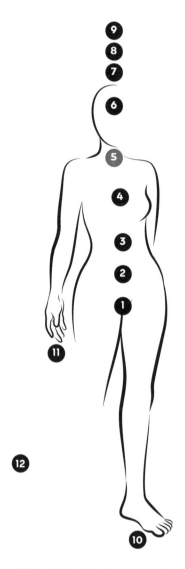

THE TWELVE-CHAKRA SYSTEM

Among chakra-ologists, the blue of the fifth chakra is often described as anything from sky blue to turquoise, although an individual's specific shade of blue can be unique to them.

Psychologically, blue is often considered the most calming of colors. Representing stability and reliability, it is nonthreatening and is preferred for situations calling for serenity and self-assurance. In fact, many studies show that blue can reduce your heart rate. It is great for office decor because people are most productive when surrounded by blue. It is also one of the least appetizing colors, however, to the point that weight-loss experts often suggest eating off a blue plate. It seems that in nature, blue is the color of poison or food spoilage. That means our biology doesn't invite us to reach for blue foods.[2]

Interestingly, blue is one of the rarest of colors in nature. In fact, blue flowers are produced by less than 10 percent of the 300,000 flowering plant species. That's because it's hard for nature to make the types of molecules that enable us to see blue.

The seeing of colors is an interesting activity. When you perceive a sparkling sapphire or a bright blue blossom, you

2 Kendra Cherry, "The Color Blue: Meaning and Color Psychology," *Verywell Mind*, February 20, 2024, https://www.verywellmind.com /the-color-psychology-of-blue-2795815.

CHAPTER ONE

aren't really perceiving blue. Rather, the object is absorbing white light. Whatever doesn't stay absorbed is reflected. You can only see a blue subject in nature—for example, a blue flower—because the red part of the spectrum is absorbed by the plant and the blue is reflected.[3]

You'll learn ways to interact with colors to refresh and boost your fifth chakra in chapter 12.

SOUND OF THE FIFTH CHAKRA

According to the ancient Hindus, each chakra emits a unique tone. Called *bija*, seed, or master sounds, they are often used as mantras. A mantra is a sound that activates a meditative state. When a one-syllable bija is uttered aloud or even focused on internally, it simultaneously awakens and purifies the chakra.

In Sanskrit, the bija of your fifth chakra is *Ham*, which sounds like "hum." To deepen into your fifth chakra, you can hum or chant its specific bija to invite healing and calm. In chapter 11 you'll acquire even more knowledge about using this mantra and other fifth chakra tones.

In addition, modern spiritual circles often link the note G to the fifth chakra. It is the logical progression from the tones associated with the lower chakras, which start with

---

3 Mindy Weisberger, "Why is the color blue so rare in nature?" *Live Science*, September 6, 2021, https://www.livescience.com/why-blue-rare-in -nature.html.

chakra one as C and then move up the ladder (second, D; third, E; fourth, F) until we get to G.

Seed syllables are associated with at least one Hindu god and goddess and a seed carrier. The god most associated with the fifth chakra is Sadashiva or Ardhanarishvara, a very powerful multi-headed and multi-armed god. The goddess is Saraswati, whose name means "purity." In addition, there is a particular shakti linked with this chakra; a shakti is an aspect of the divine feminine responsible for creation. The sound carrier is a beneficent white elephant. You'll learn all about these figures later within this chapter.

PRACTICE

RESONATING WITH PURITY
THROUGH YOUR THROAT BIJA

As the center of purification, your fifth chakra is constantly cleansing incoming and outgoing data. The more closely we are aligned with spiritual truths, the clearer our communications. To practice this level of consciousness through your fifth chakra, try the following bija practice.

Make the *Ham* mantra (pronounced "hum") by first forming an oval shape with your lips. Push the air outward from your throat while concentrating on the hollow curve at your throat. Tone "hum" in various inflections and intensities as you exhale. Concentrate on the sweet and melodious sounds your voice and fifth chakra are creating. Then ask yourself to become clear about a message you really want to send into the world right now. Sing or chant that idea until it seemingly fills you utterly. Continue expressing that message until you're ready to return to your normal life, deciding internally to now embody that concept for the rest of the day.

SOUND CARRIER

Each chakra is linked with a particular being that carries or reflects the sound of that chakra. The sound carrier for your fifth chakra is the elephant Airavata, who has seven trunks and four tusks, each representing a divine quality or attribute.

This lovely, peaceful elephant is the lord of the herbivorous animals and the traveling vehicle for Indra. In Hinduism, Indra is the king of the *devas* (godlike beings) and *svarga* (heaven). He is sometimes considered smoky gray, the color of the clouds, but is more frequently depicted as white, representing purity.

Moving freely on the etheric planes, Airavata is open to the rays of the cosmos, with one of his seven trunks emanating the pure sound *ng*. This is a nasal sound that moves energy to the outermost brain cortex, which stores our life impressions. With this sound, these impressions can now be converted to wisdom and knowledge, enabling freedom from the reincarnation cycle.

LOTUS PETALS AND APPEARANCE

Most chakras are stylistically depicted with a unique number of lotus petals. In fact, lotus petals are showcased on all in-body chakras, each with their own unique coloration.

It's important to understand that the image of the lotus petal has its roots in both science and symbolism. From an energetic viewpoint, petals represent the swirling motion of a chakra.

As I've explained, each chakra functions on a band of frequencies, busily taking in, interpreting, and emanating the subtle and physical energies that resonate with its spectrum. In fact, each is continually processing the physical energies involved in exchanges among cells, organs, organ systems, fluids, sound waves, and electromagnetic fields. They also transport subtle energies that are photonic and phononic—that is, related to subatomic waves of light and sound. Their major movements create oscillations that, if shown in a photograph taken in a split second, would look like blooming lotus blossoms. The petals are basically the arms of the radiating fields of light and sound, and the number of them relates to the intensity of the oscillations those fields are making.

The metaphorical link between chakras and lotus petals is as fascinating as the energetic science. In Hinduism, a lotus symbolizes the spiritual life. Our soul, like the lotus plant, is birthed into the muddiest of waters. In the same way that the plant grows upward, so do we, pushing our way up through the stormy seas of life. Eventually, we blossom. We open to the sun. We realize our potential only because we have struggled and survived.

The resistance of the water isn't meant to harm us. In Hinduism, water is considered the *maya*, or illusion of life. It gives us the impetus we need to evolve.

In your pure nectar chakra, there are sixteen petals arranged from right to left, each representing a different one of the sixteen potentials a human can develop. These petals are often considered smoke colored or sometimes smoky purple and showcase sixteen letters that are deep red, red, or golden.

These letters also represent the sixteen vowel sounds of the Sanskrit language that are created through the movement of the chakra. I personally like the ideas of Harish Johari, a Hindu chakra expert. His version presents the vowel sounds like this: ANG, ĀNG, ING, ĪNG, UNG, ŪNG, ṚING, ṚING, ḶRING, ḶRĪNG, ENG, AING, ONG, AUNG, ANG, AHANG.[4]

---

4   Harish Johari, *Chakras: Energy Centers of Transformation* (Destiny Books, 2000), 69.

FIFTH CHAKRA SYMBOLS: THE YANTRAS

A *yantra* is a geometric diagram that serves as a representative symbol. Yantras have been used in Indian culture for over 13,000 years to aid in meditation.

Usually, the focus of a yantra is a god or goddess. The idea is that when you concentrate on a yantra symbol, you will receive a blessing from that deity. The gift might come as a healing, a message, or a manifestation. Individuals have also been known to use a yantra to keep them on the road toward meeting a creative goal or achieving their overall purpose. Ultimately, through the fifth chakra, the yantra assists you in expressing your authentic self.

The vishuddha yantra is a silver crescent within a white circle that shines like the full moon. Many perceive the crescent sitting on the tail of the symbol in the center. Within the storyline of this yantra, the moon image represents psychic energy, clairvoyance, and the ability to communicate without words.

This white moon sits in a downward-pointing, sky blue triangle surrounded by sixteen petals. The silver crescent is the lunar symbol of *nada*, the purest cosmic sound, and represents the purification provided to the yogi whose energy ascends through the chakras. The lunar phase of the moon is also about the need to rest, release, and let go.

The white, ethereal region of this yantra also features the fifth chakra's elephant sound carrier. Indra sits upon Airavata. Indra, known as the storm god, is white, has four arms, holds a noose and a goad, grants boons, and dispels fear. In his lap are the deities described in the "Ruling Goddesses" and "Ruling Gods" sections later in this chapter. It is interesting that Airavata is known for being able to bind together the clouds. That means that the mighty elephant, through his relationship with Indra, allows us to move beyond our restrictive boundaries into greater freedom.

One of the outcomes of interacting with the fifth chakra yantra is to help activate your *siddhi* powers, which are fantastical psychic aptitudes. We'll describe these types of traits in chapter 3.

GROSS ELEMENT

In many religions, especially those also considered spiritual medical systems, matter is composed of several different elements. In most Eastern religions, it is thought that there are four or five basic elements. Always named are earth, water, fire, and wind (or air). Some systems also endorse a fifth element, space; it is also called ether or *akasha* and is the element of the fifth chakra.

Akasha combines the essence of the other four elements but is without color, smell, taste, touch, or form. It is stillness, emptiness, and endlessness. As the quintessential element, it is the spiritual energy that links all things and beings together, bringing harmony and balance to existence.

Color of the Gross Element

At one level, akasha, the gross or major element of this chakra, is the space between and within matter, as clear as a sky without clouds. In the West, this void-related element is often depicted as blue; in the Tantric system, it is a smoky purple. Both are suitable hues for the throat chakra and its relationship with clear communication.

PRACTICE

BECOME AS BLUE AS ETHER

Blue is the color most often ascribed to the ether/akasha element. Like the waters deep under the seas, this blue is unaffected by the storms of life. Whether we perceive the ether as blue, turquoise, or smoky purple, it guarantees ease and awareness.

To incorporate the truth of blue, begin by breathing deeply. Let your mind quickly run through any sources of agitation that are disturbing you right now. Allow whatever is jagged and frenetic to surface as you bring your consciousness into the middle of your throat chakra.

Next, imagine that a soothing mist begins to emanate from this inner chamber. Azure, smoky, indigo, cloudy, or clear streams of blue effortlessly ripple from and beyond your throat chakra until they encompass the entirety of your physical and subtle bodies. What was frenzied and frantic is now softened and soothed.

Anytime you want to, return to an everyday stance. Know, however, that for the next few hours, every time you breathe, this ethereal vapor will continue to fill you with bliss and peace while transforming the toxins of your mind and body into useful natural energy.

PREDOMINANT SENSE AND SENSE ORGAN

Each of your seven in-body chakras is linked with a sense and a sensory organ. It is vital to understand this concept.

Chakras are universally explained as subtle energy organs. This depiction can lead us to assume that they are only psychic in nature; even though we've already established that they are based in the body, we might imagine them as only ethereal. However, every chakra runs a certain sense and the physical organ linked to it. The sense associated with your throat chakra is your hearing, quite appropriately, and the sense organ is your ears.

Hearing is a complicated sense. Physically, it involves taking in sound waves through the ear apparatus, bones, and skin. Vibrations transferred via the body and then into your brain are interpreted by your internal programming, or related memories and beliefs. When your fifth chakra is evolved, it can hear *and* listen. This means it can intuit the meanings of the messages between words, the pauses in a poem, the cadence of a song, and the silence between sounds.

I encourage you to try an experiment with your fifth chakra sense and its sense organ. For an entire day, pay attention to the vibrations cloaked in the messages, sounds, or noises that arise in your mind or are heard by your ears. See what happens if you decide to discern between what seems false and true, and act accordingly.

ACTION ORGAN

All in-body chakras are associated with an action organ, a bodily area that transfers physical energy into the chakra so it can assume its highest functions. Regarding the fifth chakra, the action organ is the mouth.

Your mouth serves many functions. It enables you to eat and drink and thereby nourish yourself. It protects the soft tissues of the fifth chakra. It is also your vehicle for expression, enabling you to share what is occurring deep within you and your other chakras. And when you keep your mouth closed, whatever you are thinking is contained.

VITAL BREATH

In Hinduism, there is a unified vital life force called *prana*. Prana animates all living beings, pulsing through our subtle bodies and our physical structures. Considered a subtle energy, it also impacts all levels of the body, enabling activity but also supporting the unconscious tasks keeping us alive, such as automatic breathing and food digestion. Meaning "primary energy" in Sanskrit, prana is also called "spirit breath," "breath of life," and the "vital principle." The most obvious manifestation of prana is the breath.

There exist five different types of pranas, which are also called *vayus* or winds. Your fifth chakra is linked with one of these winds: *Udana* is an upward-moving breath, directing the flow of prana from the lower to the higher forms of consciousness. It is a radiant force that shifts your mind from waking to deep sleep and to the highest planes of existence after death. At a mundane level, it governs the throat, brain, and face, and it fuels how we perceive and react to our surroundings.

ATTRIBUTE

An attribute is a quality. A quality often links what seem to be positive and negative characteristics, making it our job to find the middle ground. This is certainly true regarding the fifth chakra's attribute, which is embodied by its sound carrier, the white elephant.

The attribute of this chakra is the intersection of ego and unity. Ego leads to individuality, and the truth of unity merges us with oneness. When we strike a balance between separateness and connection, we might find ourselves enjoying life the same way an elephant does. We know ourselves as a member of a herd as well as a force unto ourselves.

RULING GODDESSES

Two goddesses relate to the fifth chakra. Governing it is Saraswati. The goddess of music, art, wisdom, and learning, Saraswati offers her followers a celestial river of healing. She is usually depicted with four arms, which symbolize the mind, intellect, intelligence, and ego. To show that she is grounded as well as a carrier of higher knowledge, she sits in a lotus pose. She can be called upon to ignite and sustain your creative spark. Clad in white garments, she is as white as the moon. She is quite beautiful and holds many objects, including a book that represents knowledge.

If you want to offer a chant to Saraswati, *Om Aim Saraswatyai Namaha* translates to "Salutations to Saraswati." Simply utter "Oom eye-m suh-ruhs-vuht-yeye nuh-muh-huh" while focusing on the wisdom you seek to gain.

The shakti or divine feminine energy related to your fifth chakra is Shakini. Shown as shining white or yellow, she is five-faced, three-eyed, and four-armed. She holds several objects; depictions vary, but her items may include a noose, goad, book, bow and arrow, or trident. She is seated on a red lotus and helps bestow higher knowledge and all the siddhis, as well as mastery of the five elements and psychic communication.

RULING GODS

Above the *bindu*, a spiritual point above the mantra on the yantra, is Ardhanarishvara. Key gods and goddesses are often depicted in many forms; in this embodiment, the right side of Ardhanarishvara's body represents the part of him that is Shiva, the destroyer and restorer. As such, he is pictured as white. His left side is Parvati, a version of Shakti, the divine feminine, colored golden. Ardhanarishvara is androgynous and encourages us to blend our masculine and feminine aspects. He is five-faced, three-eyed, and ten-armed, and he holds a trident, a chisel or ax, a sword, the *vajra* or thunderbolt, fire, a snake, a bell, a goad, and a noose. He makes the gesture for dispelling fear.

RULING PLANET

The in-body chakras are associated with a ruling planet. The fifth chakra is managed by Mercury, the planet of mental activity and learning. Its energy supports our aesthetic capabilities and general creativity, also allowing us to come up with pragmatic solutions to our problems.

RELATED AURIC FIELD

The auric field for the fifth chakra is the fifth auric field. I will describe it in terms of my twelve-chakra system.

The fifth auric field is found atop the fourth auric field outside of the physical body, or about two feet away from the skin. Underneath the fourth field is the third layer, the second layer, and then the tenth auric field, which operates as a double for the body. Below this field is your first auric layer, which lies within the skin and outward to about an inch and a half around the entire body.

Your fifth field is regulated by the programs stored inside your fifth chakra. These are a composite of the beliefs about communication you inherited from your ancestors and those brought into your current body by your soul. Additional ideas are formulated during your childhood and throughout the rest of your life. Many of your ruling ideas have also been absorbed from your culture and environment. Your fifth auric field serves as a filter that screens external subtle information and decides which data is shared with the world. As you progress into a state of higher awareness and conscientiousness, the fifth auric field responds accordingly. After a while, you will only pay attention to concepts and messages that are good for you, and similarly will only offer messages to others that reinforce their well-being also.

YOUR SECONDARY FIFTH CHAKRAS

As promised, within this section is more information about the golden nectar I've been telling you about.

There are several so-called secret chakras linked to the higher chakras, many of these to vishuddha. The *lalana*, also called the *talu* or *talana,* lies at the base of the nasal orifice, just above the throat at the backside of the palate. As well, the *bindu visarga* is affiliated with the top of the brain but found toward the back of the head. This is the soft spot just under the skull where Hindu monks often retain a tuft of hair. Along with your fifth chakra, these two chakras form a triangle.

Your seventh chakra, which is your most spiritual center and found at the top of the head, emits the nectar that collects in the bindu visarga when you have reached an advanced level of emotional and spiritual development. This chakric name means "falling of drops." Mentioned several times in this chapter, this nectar is so powerful that it has been said to help yogis survive for forty days while buried. If your fifth chakra is not sophisticated enough—if you are failing to embrace and live by truth—the nectar is said to drop down to the first chakra and cause degeneration.

Lalana, which means both "female energy" and "tongue," is considered a secret chakra because you can only learn how to meditate upon it from a guru.

You have already been interacting with your higher palate, and I propose that many of the concepts and practices in the second half of this book will even more completely prepare you to benefit from your own golden nectar.

Lalana's description differs from one text to another. According to the Saubhagya Lakshmi Upanishad, it has twelve bright-red petals. Other texts suggest it has sixty-four silvery white petals and a bright-red pericarp called the *ghantika*, within which is an area of moon energy called *chandra kala*. It is from this source that the nectar is said to ooze.

Lalana's sixty-four petals are also said to house sixty-four powerful yoginis. These yoginis can serve as our magical teachers. By learning from and practicing with them, we can develop eight distinct siddhis, or superpowers.

Lalana is also associated with twelve nadis, which enable a yogi to gain all knowledge. There are Sanskrit letters linked to these nadis, and these are sometimes duplicated. The letters related to the lalana nadis are ha, sa, ksha, ma, la, va, ra, ya, ha, sa, kha, and phrem.

Under the lalana is the *golata* chakra. While lalana is placed inside the soft upper palate, golata is found on the uvula, at the back of the throat. Together, these chakras are often called the "Mouth of God." There couldn't be a more fitting label for the chakras and processes involved in your most beautiful communication vehicle, your pure nectar chakra.

CELESTIAL PLANE OF THE FIFTH CHAKRA

There are a variety of chakras and planes of existence that are located below your first chakra. These cosmic realms are called *lokas*, and they appear as luminous spheres. Each is a level of existence that we must eventually embrace as a mental state to achieve a higher state of consciousness. The one related to your fifth chakra is the *jana loka*. It is thought to be the plane of creativity, which consists of the human realm and liberated souls. Some yogis believe that if the soul doesn't learn the lessons of the fifth chakra, it will live in the jana loka until rebirth.

SUMMARY

Your lovely blue fifth chakra, core to communication and truth, is rightly the home of akasha, the ethereal element. Found in your throat and your cervical vertebrae, it manages the physical functions in this area. Its action organ is your mouth and its sensory organ your ears, which govern hearing. It is here that you reach the jana loka, the plane of creativity, and can summon your most truthful nature.

Symbolized by a moon-evoking yantra, this sixteen-petaled chakra can help you uncover the depths of your soul, which can then discern truth from not-truth. Its bija, *Ham*, is carried by a mighty elephant, and developmental strides are supported by the goddess Saraswati and the shakti named Shakini, in addition to the god Sadashiva in the form of Ardhvanarisvara. With plenty of help from the ruling planet of Mercury, your goal is to attain the level of enlightenment necessary to evoke the production of a golden nectar called *amrita*. It is this luscious fluid that drops from the seventh chakra into the fifth chakra through a secondary chakra called lalana. When you're operating from a place of true fifth chakra consciousness, this nectar will burn out your bodily toxins and further enable you to express your truths.

Gather all the fascinating knowledge you've gleaned about your fifth chakra and take a deep breath. We're going to embark on a journey into this chakra's body wisdom.

2

THE PHYSICAL SIDE

From the time we're young, we're all about interacting with the physical world. Food, clothing, and toys eventually give way in importance to housing, cars, and furniture. No matter where we are in this graduated sequencing, the body remains all important. Just as the fifth chakra must be healthy if you are to be physically healthy, the reverse is also true. That is why this chapter is devoted to the physicality of your fifth chakra.

Covered here are descriptions of the physical reach of your fifth chakra, including the organs, bodily areas, and functions involved. I'll even let you know what might occur if this chakra isn't healthy. You'll find that the golden nectar I keep mentioning is also partially rooted in the physiology of this chakra.

As you become educated in the physical nature of your fifth chakra, know that you're giving yourself an amazing gift. You're renewing your physiological relationship with yourself, the earth, and the cosmos.

OVERVIEW OF THE FIFTH CHAKRA'S PHYSICAL REACH

Your fifth chakra is anchored in your throat area, including both the front and back of the neck. Think of how often you rely on this bodily region for your well-being. Here are the parts of the body you need to breathe, eat, speak, pivot your head, regulate certain hormones, and even think.

From a spinal point of view, this chakra is anchored in the cervical nerve plexus and the seven cervical vertebrae, labeled C1 to C7. Also within this spinal area sits the laryngeal nerve plexus, associated with your larynx. Commonly called the voice box, this key to communication is connected to muscles and ligaments in your neck between C3 and C7.

The major endocrine gland linked to your fifth chakra is the thyroid. This gland controls the way your body uses energy and is the topic of an entire section in this chapter.

AREAS OF THE BODY MANAGED

Your fifth chakra is a very busy region of your body. The range of body parts it manages includes your neck, ears, jaw, teeth, mouth, trachea, larynx, pharynx, thyroid gland, parathyroid glands, cervical vertebrae, esophagus, and upper shoulders. Many of the brain's functions related to hearing are the province of the fifth chakra. This chakra is also associated with the all-important vagus nerve.

Right under the back of your skull is a set of twelve paired cranial nerves that emanate from the back of your brain. Most of them exchange electrical signals between your brain, face, eyes, and neck, helping you taste, see, smell, hear, and feel. One cranial nerve in particular, the vagus, is longer than the others and runs through many parts of your body, impacting regions including your tongue, throat, heart, and digestive system. On an energetic basis, the vagus winds through bodily areas monitored by the chakras. It also links what are known as your three brains.

Your *head brain* stores beliefs associated with many of your mental and physiological functions and processes thoughts. Your *heart brain* invites higher awareness. Then there is your enteric nervous system, also called the *gut brain*.

The gut brain controls your digestion but also most of your feelings, reactions to stress, and immune system. It is made of a web of neurons deep within your digestive system that connect to your central nervous system. It is often considered to be socially programmed, which means that it holds ideas that determine your stress-based reactions. These programs include chemical codes or psychological ideas inherited from your ancestry or enacted by your family of origin during childhood. They are also based on your own life experiences, cultural observations, religious observances, and more. Basically, these programs are templates that determine your reactions to stimuli, both internal and external. Most of the dominant messages originate in the gut brain and flow upward to your head brain. This neurological conduction occurs with your fifth chakra, based in the neck, serving as a gateway to this flow of neurological impulses.

If the physical structures or functions of your fifth chakra are compromised, the transport of data between the body and the head can also be seriously impacted, leading to issues ranging from physical illnesses to emotional problems.

ASSOCIATED GLAND: YOUR THYROID AND PARATHYROID

Your thyroid is the main endocrine gland of the fifth chakra. It is a butterfly-shaped organ located in the lower neck, just below the Adam's apple and along the front of the trachea. It has two side lobes that are bridged in the middle.

The thyroid is rich in blood vessels and nerves and secretes important bodily hormones. The main thyroid hormone is thyroxine, or T4. Along with the other thyroid hormones, T4 influences metabolism, growth and development, and body temperature. Thyroid problems are widespread and include hypo- and hyperthyroidism, Graves' disease, Hashimoto's disease, digestive and weight problems, and exhaustion.

The four parathyroid glands are also associated with the fifth chakra, although they are secondary in importance. These glands are located next to the thyroid, and while their names would suggest otherwise, the thyroid and parathyroid do not interrelate biologically. The four glands make a parathyroid hormone that controls the level of calcium in our blood and bones. Calcium determines the production of electric currents along our nerves, enabling our nerves to talk with each other.

RELATED PHYSICAL STRESSORS, PROBLEMS, AND ILLNESSES

Health issues involving the fifth chakra can be varied. I have already sprinkled a few maladies in this chapter, such as problems that arise when the vagus nerve is compromised. Additional challenges include asthma, bronchitis, mouth ulcers, thyroid dysfunctions, sore throat, tongue problems, laryngitis, ear infections, hearing issues, mouth problems, teeth and gum issues, tinnitus, tonsillitis, neck issues, upper arm pain, hay fever, and temporomandibular joint (TMJ) disorders. The pure nectar chakra is also complicit in shoulder and neck issues.

A CASE FOR BIOLOGICAL GOLDEN NECTAR

As the story has been shared for thousands of years, when one reaches a certain state of development, a golden nectar, called amrita in the Hindu literature, drops from the seventh chakra through the palate of the mouth. This half-poison, half-balm now percolates within the fifth chakra, specifically stored within the lalana, one of the fifth chakra's secondary chakras that was discussed in the last chapter. If you have cleansed your fifth chakra and have decided to operate from a truthful place, the poison is negated. In fact, all toxins will continually be eradicated from the body. If not, the nectar will remain venomous and drop into a lower chakra and negatively impact your health.

On an even more precise biological level, this nectar seems to be made of actual biological substances. During a major kundalini awakening—another term used for an accelerated growth in spirituality—the spine becomes more ionized. This means that its fluids become supercharged, full of enriched ions (charged particles), endorphins (feel-good hormones), and more. This fluid circulates through the spine, organs, and tissues, as well as through the brain. Upon spreading, this electrified fluid relaxes the body and sends wave pulses into the neurons. Cellular membranes respond, and the entire body becomes more functional. Even more alterations are made within the brain in response or perhaps even precede some of the spinal fluid alterations.[5]

There are several organs in the brain that are involved in the biological renderings of the enlightenment process. Modern physicians of the soul are now postulating that a brain organ called the caudate nucleus might play as valid a role as does the pineal gland, which has long been known as an enlightenment organ (I'll discuss the pineal a bit further on). On the physical level, the caudate nucleus is part of the basal ganglia and plays a role in learning and memory. We have two caudate nuclei, which are C-shaped bodies near the center of the brain and astride the thalamus. Each is housed in one of the two hemispheres of the brain.

The left caudate, along with the thalamus, regulates communication skills and tells us how to respond to stimulation. Both caudate nuclei store memories and transmit

5   Carol A. Seger and Corinna M. Concotta, "The Roles of the Caudate Nucleus in Human Classification Learning," *The Journal of Neuroscience* 25, no. 11 (March 16, 2005), https://doi.org/10.1523/JNEUROSCI .3401-04.2005; Viola Petit Neal and Shafica Karagulla, *Through the Curtain* (Devorss and Co., 1993); Bruce Crosson, *Subcortical Functions in Language and Memory* (Guilford Press, 1992), 47.

worry and concern inside the brain. They are also the locations of 80 percent of the brain's receptor sites for dopamine, a neurotransmitter that causes euphoria. And when the caudate nuclei are appropriately stimulated, they seem to either set off or at least play a major role in other hormonal alterations that lead to the release of the golden nectar as well as psychic experiences.[6]

Before rounding out our suppositions about the physicality of the Hindus' golden nectar and the role played by the fifth chakra, I'm going to briefly fill you in on events that occurred while you were a very small child.

One of the hormones clinically linked to states of higher awareness is dimethyltryptamine (DMT). Most commonly, it is described as a hormone produced by the pineal gland, which is the main endocrine gland of your seventh chakra. It is known for stimulating psychic sensations, hallucinations, and out-of-body experiences. However, it is naturally made in many bodily tissues as well as in plants and animals.

Known as the spirit molecule in a form sometimes called *meta*tonin, it is found in high concentrations in the blood of children until about age three. It is produced in a developing embryo in the first physical location of the pineal gland, which is at the back of the throat.

---

6   Viola Petit Neal and Shafica Karagulla, *Through the Curtain* (Devorss and Co., 1993); Bruce Crosson, *Subcortical Functions in Language and Memory* (Guilford Press, 1992), 182–83.

That's right. We're talking about your fifth chakra.

After a while, the pineal gland moves upward through what is going to become the palate on the roof of the mouth and into the center of the brain. However, metatonin-induced experiences after the age of three, such as those that occur through meditation, sacred medicines, near-death experiences, and other events, restimulate this specific type of DMT[7] that can be called the nectar of sublime awareness.

It might be decades before we fully understand the physiological alterations that occur with enlightenment or lead up to it. We do know, however, that the fifth chakra energetically performs vital tasks at many stages of development, and that certainly seems to include playing physical roles.

SUMMARY

Your pure nectar chakra has been known as the center of communication for seemingly forever. It is also important in creating and sustaining your physical health.

Encompassing all biological functions in the neck region, it governs bodily areas including your mouth, teeth, gums,

7   Panche Bozhikov, "Metatonin Research: The Pineal Gland and the Chemistry of Consciousness," https://www.scribd.com /document/481558261/Metatonin-Research.

jaw, tongue, cervical vertebrae, parathyroid, hearing apparatus, and its major endocrine gland, the thyroid. It is also
linked with your vagus nerve, which manages your reactions to stress.

Many life problems are involved in fifth chakra dysfunctions, from hormonal challenges to TMJ. The good news is
that when the physiology associated with this subtle energy
is healthy, so are many components of your life—which
might include the chemical changes related to living in an
enlightened way. Overall, if you support your fifth chakra's
mechanics, this chakra will support you.

Now get ready for the psychological and spiritual qualities
of your fifth chakra.

3

OF THE PSYCHE AND THE SOUL

In this chapter, you'll learn all about the psychology of your fifth chakra. This is a very soul-based undertaking, as the original meaning of the word *psychology* is formed from the words *psyche*, or "soul," and *logos*, or "study." That means this chapter is about how your soul relates to your pure nectar chakra.

You could also call this a spiritual approach to your throat chakra. To be spiritual is to be "full of spirit." Your own spirit is the essence that you are, have always been, and always will be. What more suitable approach to your fifth chakra than the ultimate knowledge: knowledge of your authentic self?

Get ready to become educated about the multifaceted growth that is possible through your fifth chakra.

In a nutshell, I'll be covering the psychological impact of this dynamic energy center, including descriptions of its overarching psychological profile and what occurs with psychological damage. Sweetening this chapter's mixture will also be in-depth discussions about the age at which this chakra activates, the archetypes associated with it, and the different intuitive aptitudes available through it. Interspersed exercises will accelerate your ability to enhance all facets of your life with truth and clarity.

OVERARCHING PSYCHOLOGICAL IMPACT

The general psychological benefit relating to your fifth chakra is the development of higher levels of awareness and the ability to communicate them effectively. This statement applies to all modes of communication and to receiving, interpreting, and sending data.

Many life events encourage us to develop both pragmatic and expanded states of consciousness, as well as a facility with language (and silence). No matter our station in life, we are all presented with ongoing opportunities to develop and test our personal ethics in relation to expression.

Now, it's not as if the Divine is wearing a judge's robe and is ready to hammer you when you make a mistake in communicating. Rather, every soul is tasked with communicating authentically from value-based philosophies and standards. It's not always easy to do. We all find ourselves spouting off nonsense instead of facts, yelling when we ought to listen, or lying instead of telling the truth. The teaching tool—the yardstick we can use to self-evaluate and make better choices in the future—is guilt.

Most of us don't like feeling guilty, which may be described as a bothered sensation in our gut. However, it's not the same as shame, which is the belief that we're bad. Guilt stems from our conscience, which invites evolution. The voice of guilt says, "You didn't do this right. Do better next time." Thus we are coaxed into behaving in a manner more suitable to our true self.

There are a lot of nuances involved in creating clear and conscious communication. We must continually decide what to voice and what not to; whether to express a need or keep quiet; what music matches our mood or if we would rather sing. Through our pure nectar chakra, we are invited to learn how to be in our own truth with all forms of communication, whether orating, singing, rapping, writing, uttering, asking, refusing, or any other form of articulation.

Lies can easily pollute this center. If we too frequently deceive ourselves or someone else, or fail to point out others' lies, it becomes harder to speak honestly. We then more easily turn angry, resentful, regretful, or evasive. A major psychological and spiritual learning related to the fifth chakra is self-responsibility. Ultimately, we are responsible for filtering communication in an accountable fashion.

The beliefs affecting this chakra's functioning often involve ideas like "I'll never get what I want," "It's dangerous to speak up for myself," or "No one cares what I think anyway." We can also adopt dogma from the other side of the coin, such as "If I don't push, I won't get my needs met," "The louder I am, the more likely I'll win," or "I must be right." Underneath malignant concepts such as these lies is usually a lack of awareness or a fear of being punished or rejected. Unfortunately, these types of inaccurate assumptions can proliferate, leading to anything from gossiping to emotional congestion.

One of the key teaching tools we face within the psychological landscape of the fifth chakra is our karma. The term *karma* is batted around frequently in spiritual circles. Too often it is interpreted as cause and effect—like, if you harmed someone else in a past life, they will hurt you in this one. That is not a true definition of karma. Rather, karma is a composite of the teachings about love that we have yet to acquire and fully embrace. For instance, if you speak in a way that is self-degrading, such as by constantly belittling yourself, you haven't gained the ability to love yourself.

In contrast, *dharma* consists of the knowledge that we have already gained—and live by—regarding love. In the end, the fifth chakra path is one of transforming karma into dharma and continuing to joyfully express dharma through our communications. For instance, once you learn how to love yourself, you will be kind to yourself, and probably others, in word and deed. Anytime you pause before you talk, refrain from hurtful criticism, or speak honestly with kindness, you are revealing the evolved state of your soul. Anytime you share what is genuinely on your heart or understand that a cruel person is really in pain, you are enacting the true nature of your soul.

Upon espousing the lessons of this chakra, the mind can stop causing problems. Supreme reasoning from your own higher self and spiritual guidance can overcome the negative emotions everyone struggles with. You can essentially start accessing all five planes of *jnana,* or awareness, and balance all your pranas (see page 34). When needed, you will receive divine guidance and become *chitta*: free from the fetters of the world.

CHAKRA ACTIVATION

Every chakra activates at a different development stage between infancy and adulthood. Now, this doesn't mean that your chakras materialize at a certain age; you were born with an intact chakra system. All your chakras are functional all the time, although some might be innately weaker than others. The reasons for this are varied and can include issues transferred in from past lives, your ancestors, your family of origin, and your own natural proclivities. Some weaknesses aren't really that; they are personal. For instance, if you're aiming to become a football player in this lifetime, you'll require a different set of chakras than if you're on track to become a computer programmer.

At any rate, every chakra dominates during a certain time range. In that period, it engages the programming already present and acquires new knowledge, which it stores and transforms into beliefs. That process also involves the related auric field, which will continue reflecting the codes within its corresponding chakra. Before the current, in-vogue chakra flips to the next one in line, the result is a complex set of psychological constructs that will continue to percolate and permeate.

Much of this programming is beneficial. Some is not. In relation to your fifth chakra, its most plastic period occurs between the ages of six and a half and eight and a half. Considered middle childhood, this span of time encompasses huge milestones. School becomes increasingly important, as do the friendships that are being formed. A child is learning important life skills, especially those related to social interactions and physical self-care.

During this stage, a child grows more independent from their family. They begin to think about the future while developing various communication abilities. A short list includes improvements in speaking, writing, reading, and everything from formulating philosophical concepts to attuning to specific types of music. Sadly, many situations can cause developmental delays. These include a lack of education, judgments about learning styles, insufficient support from parents or guardians, and negative messages from home, school, or the world at large.

From a chakra point of view, the fifth chakra turns on after the fourth chakra has had its day in the sun (ages four and a half to six and a half). This means that the maturity of the fifth chakra is at least partially impacted by the healthiness of fourth chakra relationship programming. The fourth chakra's love-based capabilities are built upon the personal power and thought forms that evolved when the third chakra awakened (ages two and a half to four and a half). In turn, the third chakra's wisdom is an outgrowth of the emotional and creative senses activated when the second chakra is strongest (ages six months to two and a half years). Underneath this is the first chakra, which represents physical safety and security needs (in utero to six months of age). We are ever moving, growing, pruning, and changing, and by the time we've entered our fifth chakra developmental platform, innumerable psychological constructs have already been laid, brick by brick.

PSYCHOLOGICAL FUNCTIONS

The easiest way to summarize the psychological functions of your fifth chakra is to compare them with the same regarding your third chakra. You do not need to have perused the third chakra book to relate to this contrasting dialogue. Rather, my discussion just might clear up a lot of questions you have about the basic differences between concepts such as thoughts and principles, data and philosophies.

In general, the third chakra, which percolates in your solar plexus area, is in charge of thoughts, whereas the fifth chakra manages principles. Understanding this distinction will explain the truly elevated psychological potential of your fifth chakra.

Thoughts are important. They are opinions or perceptions that enable us to create and follow through on plans. Ultimately, the way we perceive and organize thoughts determines how successful we are in life.

In the body, thoughts are real. They have shape and explain a subject because they are formed from neurological firings. That makes them physical—but not necessarily true. Something can be concrete but inaccurate, conclusive but not beneficial, important but useless.

Within the fifth chakra we must assess all assumptions according to the principles they lead to. A *principle* is a fundamental truth or proposition that serves as the foundation for a system of beliefs or thoughts. At baseline, a principle determines how you are to accomplish something and under what conditions. The fifth chakra will analyze third chakra data via the higher emotional assessments made possible within the heart chakra—the ladder rung between the third and fifth chakras—and in comparison to the higher truths available through the more spiritual chakras, which lie above it. Essentially, it is deciding what to put energy into and what not to—and what to share and what not to—based on more idealistic philosophies than we engage in the lower chakras.

For example, your fifth chakra will hold a message against a higher standard like love. It will toss aside individual ideas, beliefs, or thoughts that aren't aligned with principles supporting loving behavior and outcomes. It's far easier and quicker to make communication decisions based on overarching principles than on individual thoughts or opinions. Toward that end, the next practice will enable you to clarify a few of the principles most vital to your well-being.

PRACTICE

COMPOSE YOUR PERSONAL PRINCIPLES

One way to turn up the dimmer switch on the quality of pure nectar chakra communications is to clarify a few of your fundamental principles. You will then be invited to employ these in making decisions regarding your communication.

Gather a pen and paper, then isolate yourself in a quiet place. You might select an environment in nature that helps you feel serene and clear-headed. Breathe deeply, take a few minutes to settle your body and mind, and request that these aspects of self merge into your soul. Then bring your consciousness into the center of your fifth chakra and review the following list of spiritual qualities. You may also add constructs of your own.

- » authentic
- » calm
- » compassionate
- » creative
- » disciplined
- » empathic
- » flexible
- » forgiving
- » grateful
- » humble

- » loving
- » peaceful
- » purposeful
- » respectful
- » self-reliant
- » tender
- » wise

Select two or three of these virtues that resonate with your true self. Then weave these into a single principle by filling in the blanks in these two sentences (it's okay to use only one quality):

> *I will make decisions about all forms*
> *of communication based on this/these*
> *spiritual qualities:* _____
>
> *I define the meaning of this term/these*
> *terms this way:* _____

Now apply this ethic to all your communication decisions and feel your personal agency expand.

PSYCHOLOGICAL DEFICIENCIES
IN AN UNHEALTHY FIFTH CHAKRA

Deficiencies in this energy center can lead to any of the physical conditions described in the last chapter, as well as psychosomatic challenges related to communication. One problem is throat tension, which can block our ability to speak or express—and be caused by such a blockage. Teeth grinding is a common symptom of anxiety or fear of speaking, and neck pain is often related to withholding your own truth or believing in others' falsehoods. You can also become too precise or overregulated in your approach to speech, writing, or other forms of expression.

Sometimes fifth chakra psychological disturbances lead to excesses, like talking too much or too loudly. This can be a sign of being too concerned about what others might be thinking or the belief that unless we are obnoxious, no one will pay attention. Almost any sort of fifth chakra psychological challenge can cause stuttering or the inability to be understandable.

At the extreme end, compulsive behaviors often can be linked to fifth chakra problems. It's not uncommon to deal with major confusion by overeating or incessant chewing, even chewing on pencils. Smoking and other compulsive mouth-related behaviors can indicate that it's time to take a deep dive into the programs held within the fifth chakra to create a more confident and principled approach to life.

PSYCHOLOGICAL STRENGTHS IN THE HEALTHY FIFTH CHAKRA

Let yourself imagine that you are enjoying a perfectly balanced and healthy fifth chakra. This equates with your life being open to all sorts of joy, ranging from being completely expressive to quietly calm.

With a balanced fifth chakra, you'll be creative and expressive, communicate positively, listen consciously, and experience contentment. You'll find it easy to either share or withhold your truth, depending on circumstances, but you will always know what it is. In other words, you'll communicate with flow.

Spiritually, you'll be open to the guidance of others when they offer wisdom, whether it is presented through books, creative expression, words of advice, or songs on the radio. You'll also be able to provide wisdom if your soul so leads. Psychically, you'll be able to shift into the intuitive sense related to this chakra, which is called clairaudience; this ability is described further on in this chapter.

ASSOCIATED ARCHETYPES

An archetype is a template. Archetypes are models for both positive and negative behavior, and associated with the fifth chakra, there are life-enhancing and joy-detracting archetypes.

The uplifting archetype is the communicator. How apt in that this awesome prototype encourages truthfulness, relatability, open-mindedness, and honesty. Once you've embraced the communicator archetype, you become a channel for clarity and connectivity. The communicator knows that words have power, as does silence.

The shadow archetype is the silent child. This model does not reference the quietude of a clear communicator. Rather, it references the tragedy of a child who has been silenced so often that they can no longer find their voice.

A child who is judged, ignored, or shamed for their personality or ideas—even wild and carefree expressions of joy and other emotions—stops sharing. They fear rejection or punishment. Bullied, they might cease having any sense of what they even think about things. Fortunately, this type of hurt and pain can be healed.

The following short exercise will help you activate your inner fifth chakra communicator and then help free any part of you who has been silenced.

PRACTICE

ENFOLDING YOUR FIFTH CHAKRA ARCHETYPES INTO YOUR LIFE

Take a few minutes and sit alone in a quiet space. You might want to lower the lights and close your eyes; you might also want paper and pen to take notes.

Bring your awareness into the center of your fifth chakra. Breathe and be still within the calm seas of this inner sanctum. Now think of a situation in your everyday life that is calling for you to show up with clear communication. Then request that your healthy communicator present itself intuitively.

Sense how valiant and self-confident your communicator is. Imagine them in the type of clothing that reflects their confidence. Relate empathically to their boldness. Ask this communicator if there are specific messages they want to offer regarding the topic. Listen as they present melodies or lyrics, share a phrase or poem, or otherwise make their truth known. Allow yourself to enjoy this fully developed fifth chakra communicator, for you and they are the same.

Invite the communicator to step aside for a moment while you call forth a silent child. Notice how scared they are and how hard it is for them to face the situation in your mind. Look into their face and eyes as you relate to the undercurrent of their pain and suffering. Embrace this child and perceive at least one of the reasons for their repressed state. Memories of mistreatment might surface, as might feelings such as being unwanted or unrecognized.

What might have happened to this injured self if they had opened their mouth and expressed their emotions, needs, or desires? There was great harm done to this self.

Next, invite forward the communicator and introduce them to the silent child. Oh, there is so much understanding being sent from the communicator to the silent child. Watch the love flow until it fully heals that silent child and all the messages that should have been given are delivered. The truth of what is eternal—love—enables the merging of these two archetypes of yourself. They merge into your fifth chakra as a single entity, and now you can be at peace.

PERSONALITY PROFILE

Many individuals are powerfully gifted in fifth chakra capabilities. This might be your strongest chakra or one that you use a lot. No matter your personality or preference, when you are actively engaging with your fifth chakra—whether for short or extended amounts of time—you will experience yourself being all about communication. Music, reading, speaking: anything goes if you get the message across verbally.

An active fifth chakra will find you frequently opinionated and expressive; then again, you'll probably also be a good listener. Perhaps you learn by speaking aloud and even make a living through communication—from speaking to writing to playing music or offering spiritual guidance.

Of course, you can be an introverted communicator as well. I am quite shy, but I am a good teacher; when I'm speaking, I'm able to open my heart and speak with ease and joy.

THE INTUITIVE GIFT OF THE FIFTH CHAKRA

The intuitive power commonly associated with the pure nectar chakra is clairaudience, which means "clear hearing." This multifaceted gift involves obtaining psychic guidance through the back side of the fifth chakra. It is then interpreted by the brain. If it is appropriate to verbally respond or share, the front side of this chakra opens, and voilà—you are talking, singing, chanting, or otherwise making sure you're heard.

There are several forms of clairaudience. Mediumship or channeling involves communicating what external beings or forces are sharing. Guided or automatic writing occurs when outside guides enable the inscribing of messages, and certain individuals can even speak for otherworldly beings such as angels or extraterrestrials. You can use the next practice to gain an insight through your own clairaudience.

SIMPLE CLAIRAUDIENCE WITH WRITING

Focus on a subject about which you would like insight. Grab a paper and pen. In a quiet area, breathe deeply while bringing your awareness into the middle of your fifth chakra, then write down what you would like inspiration about. Phrase it in the form of a question, such as "What is the highest path for me?" or "What does spiritual guidance want me to know about this topic?" Then pause and simply write down whatever words or messages pop into your mind. Trust what you hear or whatever message comes through your hand as you write.

If what you have inscribed leads to another question, formulate that query on your paper and then take a moment before writing down a new response. Continue this process until you feel satisfied. Read everything you have written and then formulate a final statement, which you will embrace as guidance.

Take a couple of additional breaths and continue with your day when you're ready.

A FEW OTHER EXTRAORDINARY
SPIRITUAL ABILITIES

The Hindu term referring to mastering the qualities, or *tattvas*, of this chakra is *akashidharana*. At this level, a yogi holds knowledge of the four Vedas, or Hindu scriptures. It is said that when this happens, they will not perish, even if the whole universe does. They can also become *trikala-jnani*: knowledgeable about the past, present, and future.

Others of the numerous *siddhis,* or supernatural powers, associated with the fifth chakra include freedom from hunger and thirst, *laghima* (levitation), superhearing, the ability to travel through space, and mastery of the elements and the five bodily senses. With the activation of this chakra, a yogi or advanced person increases in knowledge as well as in the power of eloquence and the ability to persuade others, such as through hypnosis.

SUMMARY

As the center of all communication, your fifth chakra's psychological strengths begin and end with truth—the ability and willingness to share your own higher truth, respond truthfully to others, and bring forth conscious truths from spiritual guidance. As you hone your fifth chakra powers, including the psychic aptitude of clairaudience, you'll find yourself easily living your life in a principled way. This leads to psychological balance and an ease in responding during verbal exchanges. Otherwise, it's easy to fall prey to fifth chakra psychological imbalances, which can range from talking over others to being too shy.

Once you've come to understand the potent grace of this chakra, you can more fully activate and access it. At this point, the world transforms into a blank canvas, notation pad, musical staff paper, or other means of expression. Your soul can now formulate anything from a manuscript to a song, an ode to silence to a tapestry of words. When evolved, your pure nectar chakra helps you comprehend everything from your core ideals to methods for embodying the enlightened self.

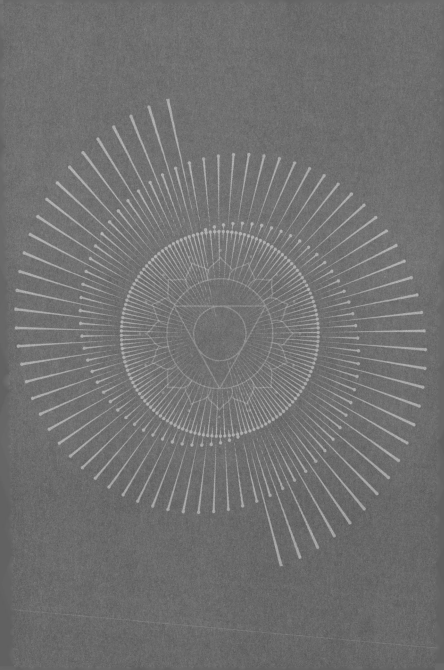

PART 2

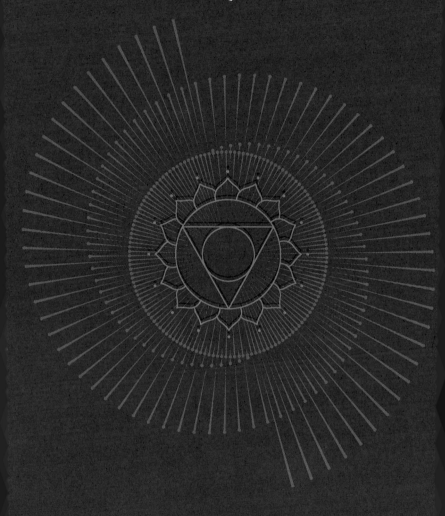

APPLYING FIFTH CHAKRA
KNOWLEDGE IN REAL LIFE

· · · · · ·

It is now time to drink from the nectar of immortality that is the fifth chakra's ultimate provision.

Welcome to part 2, the second half of your throat chakra odyssey. Within these pages you'll find myriad ways to develop your pure nectar chakra, and with that all aspects of your communication endeavors. Whether your goal is to send more loving messages into the world, better understand what others are sharing, or improve the physical or psychological functions of your throat chakra universe, everything you need to know is covered within the following chapters.

These resources for transformation are rich and varied, primarily because every chapter is written by an energy authority with specific vishuddha expertise. Drawing upon their professional know-how, each will encapsulate a particular approach to shining up your fifth chakra.

You may read and enjoy these chapters in any order. Follow your whimsy or wishes, ideas or inspirations. Maybe you want to create a foodie masterpiece to support vishuddha; the last chapter in part 2 offers throat chakra recipes from two excellent chefs. Then again, it might be timely to experience targeted yoga poses or employ color, sound, or vibrational remedies to spiff up your fifth chakra. Everything you need for fifth chakra impact is right here. As you flow through this section, you'll inevitably transcend issues lying stuck within your throat chakra and reclaim your own innate wisdom.

YOU'LL BE USING INTENTION

You've probably already heard about the benefits of using intention. Even if you haven't, it's an all-important skill that will facilitate most of the activities in part 2.

Intention is a mental state that allows you to focus on a particular scenario so it might come true. Intention can exponentially increase the benefits of the exercises in these chapters, so I will further explain the concept and offer a few pointers.

In a way, you are already an expert at intention, as it has been one of the major forces behind your accomplishments to date. The difference between daydreaming and doing, meandering and manifesting, lies in formulating and following through on an intention.

Setting an intention is a practical endeavor. It involves formulating a desire and then acting as if it is already fulfilled. This does more than engage physical energies; it also summons the all-powerful subtle energies required to shift and shape realities that support your objectives.

We've already shown that nearly 100 percent of all energy—therefore, of reality—consists of subtle energies. Adding subtle energies to an intention is like adding a wallop to a wiffle ball. No matter how softly you toss it, it's going to gain velocity. In the end, everything solid started with a strong, creative intention.

Formulating an intention is easy. There are only three steps involved in the process:

First, fashion a single-sentence statement that summarizes a desire. In fact, the practice is like creating a bit of prose or poetry in that it involves combining a noun (subject) and a verb (action) with a desire.

The caveat is that you must employ present tense. No projecting into the future or dragging the past forward. The power of an intentional declaration is its ability to convince you that the dream has already materialized.

Here are a few examples that would apply to the throat chakra:

I have completed my first book for publication.

*I easily draw on my intuition to
gain clairaudient input.*

I speak only when I have something wise to share.

Second, make sure you feel emotion when you're focusing on your intention. There isn't a goal in the world that will occur if you don't really care about it. Emotion means "energy in motion," and that's the magic sauce that enlivens even the simplest of intentions.

The third step is to make decisions—and take actions—that are logical extensions of the intention. If you are seeking to author a book, adopt habits that support the goal; you can't write a book without writing, after all.

To pep up an intention, keep it uppermost in your mind. Use it like an affirmation that you repeat internally or externally, post on your refrigerator, or put to song.

State, feel, and embody. Those are the three stages of making your dreams come true.

In preparation for the practices you'll be treated to in part 2, I'll help you design an intention right now.

Create a focus related to your pure nectar chakra. Think about the many items on your throat chakra wish list. Basically, anything centered on communication is a safe bet. Then vitalize that aspiration by forming it into a statement, like this:

> *I am in joyful communication with Spirit*
> *when I'm conversing with others.*

Now decide to keep your intention alive by repeating it as often—and in as many ways—as you can. Infuse this affirmation with emotion every time you think, say, write, or chant it. The more energy you put into owning this idea, the more potent the dream becomes. And isn't the point of your throat chakra to manifest your dreams?

4

SPIRIT ALLIES

MARGARET ANN LEMBO

There are many spirit allies—an entire support network of metaphysical assistants, in fact—ready to help you calibrate your fifth chakra, a vital center for communication.

Allies exist in many forms. Covered in this chapter are angels and archangels, animal allies, and the devic forces of essential oils. (Refer to chapter 10, my section on working with crystals, minerals, and stones, to pair them with these beings.)

Invisible allies are everywhere and available to everyone. You can access them through telepathy and mind-to-mind, heart-to-heart communication. Simply request guidance from these spirit helpers and relax into their supernatural care.

To get started, give yourself permission to feel the world with the innocence of a child. Visualize and imagine what your allies are communicating, and tune in. Let go of the notion that you are making it up, and receive the wisdom they have to share. The seen and unseen are equally real. Your allies will help improve your ability to experience your intuitive nature and inspire you with guidance and wisdom.

The throat chakra is the center where you communicate, express, and listen to others, including spiritual helpers. Improve your listening skills to hear what is being communicated, and trust your intuition. It is important to be discerning so you can connect with the spirit allies working for your highest good.

ANGELS AND ARCHANGELS

Angels and archangels are beings of light, color, and vibration. They are androgynous and invisible to the physical eyes. Both angels and archangels act and react based on your requests through your thoughts, prayers, and petitions for assistance, which are broadcast through telepathy and vibration. The major distinction between angels and archangels is that archangels are more potent and can assist with most life categories.

Angel of Animal Companions

The Angel of Animal Companions is your ally to improve your connection with the earth and activate your role as a steward and caregiver of all life. With this angel by your side, you can cultivate interspecies communication. Consider consciously dedicating time and attention to be with your furry, feathered, or scaly friends. Ask this angel to open your ears on all levels to understand interspecies communication. Take action to support a better life for all nature.

AFFIRMATIONS: I am aware of my surroundings
and intimately connect with all life in nature.
I understand what animals are communicating
to me.

Angel of Communication

Call on the Angel of Communication when you feel misunderstood or need help expressing yourself. Ask this angel to show you the steps necessary to improve your communication skills. Partner with this angel to help you find the right words to say what needs to be said and hear what others are saying. This angel helps you notice your body language and tone of voice. Allow it to help you open your connection with others on a soul-to-soul level.

AFFIRMATIONS: I speak with clarity and kindness.
I understand and am understood.

Angel of Divine Timing

This everyday angel helps you connect with the angelic realm to integrate divine orchestration into your life. The Angel of Divine Timing can shine a light so you recognize when opportunity arises and it is time to take action. Allow this spiritual helper to notice the signs and symbols along your path. Ask it to guide you in knowing when to speak up and when to say nothing.

> **AFFIRMATIONS:** Favorable opportunities present themselves often. I take action when events converge to make my life clearer and easier. I receive guidance all the time.

Archangel Azrael

Call on Azrael for comfort when you are in the depths of sorrow. This archangel comforts you and opens your consciousness to receive messages or wisdom from your loved ones on the other side. Archangel Azrael has the sacred duty of transporting souls as they depart their earthly bodies. Use this angel as an ally to heighten your awareness so you better understand the evolutionary process.

> **AFFIRMATIONS:** I open my mind and heart to receive communication from my loved ones who have passed away. I am comforted and send blessings ahead for the dearly departed.

Archangel Gabriel

Archangel Gabriel is God's chief messenger angel and was sent to various prophets, including Mohammad and Daniel. Archangel Gabriel is the Angel of the Annunciation, well known for appearing to Mother Mary to tell her of the conception of Jesus Christ. This is the same archangel that came to Zacharias, the husband of Elizabeth, who was too old to conceive, and told him she would give birth to his son, John the Baptist. Call on Archangel Gabriel for inspired advice and to help you with your intuition and inner knowing. Gabriel is known for bringing messages in dreams. Pay attention to your dreams and use the information in your waking life.

> **AFFIRMATIONS**: I receive messages in various ways all the time. Guidance comes to me in dreams and signs in my waking life. I understand the messages from the angels.

ANIMAL ALLIES

The connectedness of everything on our planet—from rocks and crystals to plants and animals—links messages and lessons from the animal kingdom to your consciousness for personal awareness and growth. There are many animal allies to help you, including bats, blue jays, cardinals, crows, dolphins, elephants, mockingbirds, parrots, and whales. Here are a few animal allies that can bring you messages and realizations on your spiritual journey.

Blue Jay

Blue Jay is an ally that helps you find the courage to use your voice to protect yourself and those you care about. Call on this bird's energy when you must speak up for yourself. When Blue Jay shows up in your life, it is a sign that you must express what needs to be said for the good of all. Be courageous and establish boundaries when necessary.

> **AFFIRMATIONS**: It is easy for me to communicate with clarity and grace. It is safe for me to set boundaries in loving ways. I deserve respect.

Cardinal

Cardinals are songbirds that establish their territory with their song. They communicate with their life mates and other birds using varying sound patterns. Turn to cardinal's vibe to help you find different tones and ways of expressing yourself. For example, try using a softer voice or a lower pitch. Look to this totem as an ally for communicating with confidence.

> **AFFIRMATIONS**: My communication skills are effective. I find the courage to express myself in healthy ways. I consciously shift the tone of my voice to garner a better result.

Crow

Crows are very good communicators. They caw loudly, which often serves as a warning to their companions that a predator is nearby. Crow is an ally for you, too, so pay attention to the crow's caw. This bird might alert you to a negative situation or influence. Crow has helped me many times throughout my life.

> **AFFIRMATIONS**: Messages come to me in many ways. I observe and am mindful. I pay attention to the guidance sent my way.

AROMATHERAPEUTIC ALLIES

The fifth chakra is all about how we communicate and express ourselves in the world, including through writing, speaking, singing, cooking, and more. Aromatherapy is the use of essential oils derived from the aromatic parts of plants in the form of oils, mists, incense, and sprays to heal physical, mental, and emotional complaints and improve your overall well-being.

Chamomile Essential Oil

Chamomile essential oil calms your nerves. Inhaling chamomile is beneficial for calming effects that help you sort out your thoughts and communicate more effectively. Chamomile helps cancel out angry, vindictive, or negative thoughts and shifts the vibration of expression. Use it to quell emotional outbursts.

> **AFFIRMATIONS**: I am calm and peaceful. I am content. I go with the flow and express myself calmly and peacefully.

> **FOR YOUR SAFETY**: Avoid if allergic to asters, daisies, chrysanthemums, or ragweed. Do not use if pregnant or nursing. Roman chamomile should be avoided in the first trimester of pregnancy.

Eucalyptus Essential Oil

Eucalyptus essential oil opens breathing passages and reduces the symptoms of cold, flu, and allergies. It has a cooling quality that is useful if you are feeling hot-headed. Inhale eucalyptus to release negative thoughts and feelings of agitation and frustration before expressing yourself; it clears intense emotions. Spray it in a mist to shift the energy of a room.

> **AFFIRMATIONS**: It is easy for me to express myself in a calm manner. My space is clear and filled with well-being.

> **FOR YOUR SAFETY**: Avoid (or use small amounts) if epileptic or in cases of high blood pressure. It may interfere with the efficacy of homeopathic remedies. Do not use if pregnant or nursing. Avoid use on children.

Ravensara Essential Oil

Ravensara essential oil can clear toxic, repetitive thoughts, creating space for higher levels of prophetic dreaming and messages from deep within yourself. Inhale it to quiet your mind and bring emotional balance. Ravensara clears congestion and is good for the respiratory system as an antiviral. It is beneficial for healthy ears, nose, and throat.

> **AFFIRMATIONS**: Dreams bring me guidance and inspiration. I have clarity of mind. My emotions are balanced.

> **FOR YOUR SAFETY**: Do not use if pregnant or nursing.

Tea Tree Essential Oil

The clean, clear aroma of tea tree essential oil is beneficial to channel higher consciousness and awaken the spiritual gift of clairaudience. The crisp aroma brings mindfulness and aids in opening a conduit for mind-to-mind communication. It is especially beneficial for relieving a sore throat, toothache, earache, or sinus conditions.

> **AFFIRMATIONS**: I receive help and guidance from the angelic realm. I am a good listener. My intuition is intact.

> **FOR YOUR SAFETY**: Possible skin irritant.

SUMMARY

Working with angels, animal allies, and essential oils will improve your fifth chakra awareness. You are never alone, so use the healing vibrations of angels and nature paired with your intentions and positive thoughts. Choose good thoughts and create a wonderful reality. Enjoy these wonderful energies.

5

YOGA POSES

AMANDA HUGGINS

Your yoga practice can yield concrete benefits for both your physical and energetic bodies. Different yoga poses target and engage specific muscles, and every muscle in the body is intricately connected to a specific chakra. As you move through the physical postures, you simultaneously facilitate energetic flow within the subtle body.

The activation of the fifth or throat chakra is facilitated by yoga poses that involve stretching and opening the neck and shoulders, thereby directly engaging the muscles associated with the throat chakra. These throat-opening poses promote flexibility and strength in the neck, creating a direct, open pathway for the flow of energy to and from the fifth chakra. Additionally, poses such as upward-facing dog and camel contribute to the activation of the throat chakra by enhancing blood circulation and stimulating the respiratory system. The fifth chakra is closely connected to the respiratory system through the regulation of breath, vocal expression, and the overall health of the throat region.

Beyond the physical aspects, yoga delves into the spiritual dimensions of the throat chakra's influence: the expression of truth and authenticity. A consistent yoga practice encourages self-awareness and mindfulness, creating a conducive environment for individuals to explore and embrace their true selves. As you cultivate mindfulness and presence on the mat, you'll find an alignment between your inner truth and external expressions, thus aligning yourself with the essence of the throat chakra.

PRACTICE

UJJAYI BREATH IN YOGA

Yoga offers a fantastic opportunity to harness deep, rhythmic breathing to conduct the flow of energy in and out of the throat chakra. This is *pranayama*, the yogic practice of breath regulation. Practices like *ujjayi*, or "victorious" breath, where breath is controlled and audibly regulated, stimulate the throat area and promote a mindful connection to the body.

Energetically, focused breathwork helps clear energetic blockages within the throat chakra, allowing for less obstructed energy flow. Physically, ujjayi breath supports your yoga practice by ensuring that you stay intimately connected to your body during particularly challenging *asanas* (poses). The controlled and audible nature of ujjayi breath serves as an anchor, grounding your awareness in the present moment; as you synchronize each movement with the rhythmic flow of breath, you cultivate a profound mind-body connection. During especially demanding yoga sequences, ujjayi breath acts as a stabilizing force, helping you manage physical exertion and preventing unnecessary strain. The audible quality of ujjayi serves as a constant reminder, allowing you to tune in to the subtleties of your body's response and make any necessary adjustments.

Ujjayi is characterized by the contraction of the glottis, creating a gentle sound resembling ocean waves or the soft whisper of the wind. Here's a step-by-step guide on how to practice this powerful breath.

> » Find a comfortable seat: Begin by sitting in a cross-legged position or assuming a yoga pose of your choice. Ensure your spine is straight, allowing for optimal breath flow.

> » Relax your body: Close your eyes and take a moment to relax your facial muscles, particularly around the jaw and throat. Allow the shoulders to soften, releasing any tension in the neck or upper body.

» Natural breathing: Start with a few rounds of natural, deep breaths.

» Constrict the back of the throat: Slightly constrict the back of your throat, creating a gentle restriction of the passage of air. This is like the sensation of fogging up a mirror with your breath.

» Inhale and exhale through the nose: Inhale deeply through the nose, allowing your breath to be smooth and consistent. As you exhale, maintain the slight constriction in the throat, producing a sound akin to the ocean or a gentle whisper.

» Repeat for a few cycles of breath: Continue this flow of inhaling and exhaling through the nose with a gentle restriction to familiarize yourself with the feel of ujjayi.

Once you feel comfortable with ujjayi in a seated position, integrate it into your yoga practice. Use it during asanas to create a rhythmic flow that synchronizes with your movements. Remember, ujjayi is a personal practice, and the sound should be soothing rather than forced. It may take some time to develop the technique, so be patient in your process of cultivating this powerful and grounding pranayama.

PRACTICE

YOGA FLOW TO
ACTIVATE THE FIFTH CHAKRA

Before immersing yourself in this yoga flow, take a mindful pause to set your intention for your practice. In the spirit of activating the pure nectar chakra, you may choose to use one of the following intentions:

» Clear expression: To open and balance the throat chakra, allowing for clear and authentic expression of your thoughts and emotions. Use the mantra "I am worthy of expressing my truth."

» Harmonious listening: To develop the capacity to listen actively and empathetically. Use the mantra "I am listening."

» Empowered self-expression: To empower yourself to express your individuality and unique voice without fear of judgment. Use the mantra "I speak my truth."

» Mindful breath and sound: Intend to use the breath to foster deeper connection to the throat chakra, creating a stronger mind-body connection. Use the mantra "I am intentional."

Holding an intention for your yoga practice will serve as a reminder of the mind-body connection and anchor you in conscious awareness of your fifth energy center. It will fortify your practice by infusing it with mindfulness, purpose, and a deliberate connection to your own personal expression.

» begin in a comfortable position

Start in any seated position that feels comfortable for your body. Place your hands on your knees. Lengthen your spine and take a few deep, natural breaths. On your exhales, focus on releasing any tension in the neck and shoulders.

» integrate ujjayi breath

Now gently constrict the flow of air as you breathe in and out through the nose. Focus on the warming sensation that ujjayi creates in the back of your throat, and tune in to the oceanic quality of the breath. As you move throughout this practice, do your best to maintain ujjayi breathing, fluidly syncing your breath and movement.

» seated neck stretches

Keeping your hands placed on your knees, tilt your head to the right so the right ear moves toward the right shoulder. Feel the lengthening of the left side of your neck and stay for three cycles of breath. Repeat on the left side. These seated neck stretches serve as a grounding and preparatory phase, setting the tone for your throat chakra–focused flow.

» move into cat/cow pose

Leave the seated position and come onto your hands and knees, with your shoulders stacked above your wrists in tabletop position. On your next inhale, arch your back, lift your tailbone, and gaze upward for cow pose, feeling a stretch along the front of your neck. Exhale, round your spine, tuck your chin to your chest, and curl your tailbone under for cat pose, feeling the stretch along the back of your neck. Repeat this flow with your breath for a few rounds, experimenting with the sensations of the neck and throat space opening and closing.

» flow into downward-facing dog

From tabletop position, lift your hips up and back, coming into an inverted V shape with your body. Press your palms and feet firmly into the mat and allow your heart to melt toward your thighs. Aim to broaden and open the chest space. Maintain ujjayi here as you take a few full, deep breaths, or you may choose to momentarily break from ujjayi breathing and take a few audible exhales, sighing or otherwise audibly releasing energy.

» assume plank pose

From downward-facing dog, come into a high push-up position, again aligning your shoulders directly over your wrists. Hold plank pose for five cycles of ujjayi breath. If the body feels challenged by the longer hold, direct more focus to the quality and sound of the breath as an anchor point. After the fifth cycle of breath, lower all the way to your belly.

» go into cobra pose

Place your hands underneath your shoulders, keeping your elbows close to the body. Inhale as you press into the palms and lift your chest off the mat, keeping the lower body grounded. Engage the throat chakra by directing your gaze forward, opening the throat and heart space. Lower down on an exhale. Repeat cobra pose three more times, syncing movement with breath.

» face up with upward-facing dog

On the next inhale, press through your palms, straightening your arms and lifting your chest and thighs off the mat. Find the same throat chakra activation that you found in cobra pose: neck and heart space open as you inhale and exhale deeply. Hold here for one full cycle of ujjayi and then return to downward-facing dog.

» achieve warrior 2 with lion's breath

From downward-facing dog, step your right foot forward in between your hands. Pivot the back foot, aligning it parallel to the back edge of the mat. On an inhale, lift the torso upright and extend the arms out to the sides parallel to the floor, palms facing down. Drop the shoulders away from the ears. Once you've settled into this pose, practice lion's breath to activate the throat chakra.

Stick out your tongue and exhale forcefully while making a "ha" sound. Feel how this powerful breath clears and opens energy in your fifth chakra. Hold the pose and practice lion's breath three more times. When you've finished, return your hands to the mat and find downward-facing dog again. Repeat warrior 2 with lion's breath on the other side, then return to downward-facing dog.

» come into camel pose

From downward-facing dog, release the knees to the mat and come to a kneeling position. Place your hands on your lower back, fingers pointing downward, and then simultaneously lift your chest and arch your upper spine. If it feels safe for your neck and throat, you may drop your head back and allow for a full expansion of the front of the throat and chest region. Otherwise, keep the chin slightly tucked and focus on lengthening the back of the neck. Stay here for three to five cycles of ujjayi. When you feel complete, tuck the chin again and gently sit back down on your heels. Breathe deeply.

» assume fish pose

Find your way onto your back. Bring your palms underneath your hips, tucking your forearms beneath your body. Lift your chest and tilt your head back slightly to emphasize the expansion of the throat chakra. Breathe deeply for three cycles of ujjayi, allowing the front of the throat to gently open and release.

» soothe into savasana

Transition from fish pose by gently lowering your back to the mat, extending your legs, and releasing your arms alongside your body with the palms facing up. Release ujjayi breathing and allow your breath to return to a natural, relaxed state. Close your eyes and rest here for at least five to ten cycles of breath. As you rest, visualize a calming blue light enveloping your body and flowing through your being.

SUMMARY

Through intentional breath control, mindful poses, and throat-opening postures like fish pose, cobra pose, and camel pose, you can open physical channels that promote greater energetic flow within the fifth chakra. The integration of pranayama with ujjayi breath also serves as a guiding force, fostering a balance between your physical and energetic body. With practice, this mind-body connection will allow you to fully unlock the potential of the throat chakra, promoting clear and authentic expression both on and off the mat.

6

BODY WISDOM

LINDSAY FAUNTLEROY

In indigenous cultures, the throat chakra holds tremendous importance. Humans evolved from oral traditions in which sacred stories were passed down from generation to generation. Many of these stories were catalogued and memorized by the community's priests and wisdom holders, becoming the foundation of divination systems that are among the world's first recordings of sacred symbols. Though they were rendered as written text much later in human history, we carry the ancestral remembrance of the power of storytelling, symbol making, myth, and sound as co-creative forces that reside in our fifth chakra.

In this chapter, I will provide several insights and practices that enable you to develop a strong and powerful throat chakra. All will employ the sacred nature of the fifth chakra as a communication portal.

THE IMPORTANCE OF THE
FIFTH CHAKRA AND WORDS

When interacting through your fifth chakra, you are essentially embracing the power and impact of words. Words have meaning, and they also have energy that is mediated by our fifth chakra.

Our ancestors understood that we live in a dynamic universe in which everything is vibration.[8] In fact, the universe is created through vibration, with the throat chakra serving as the gate between the imagined and the manifested worlds.

Through sound and vibration, ideas and inspiration come out of the invisible and intangible and into the world of substance and form. This vibration—often through its naming and speaking—is the first imprint of existence. Using our fifth chakra to express our intentions through words or art is a powerful first step in manifestation. It is also why we begin to heal when we can give voice to our pain, traumas, worries, doubts, and fears. I know that my patients have reached a powerful point in their healing when they are able to share some of the core wounds standing in the way of their wholeness that were previously unconscious. Storytelling is a powerful tool for healing,

8   Wayne Chandler, *Ancient Future: The Teachings and Prophetic Wisdom of the Seven Hermetic Laws of Ancient Egypt* (Black Classic Press, 2000).

manifesting, and transforming our experience in the physical world; thus we embody the medicine of the pure nectar chakra.

SACRED NAMING

After my daughter was born and received the divination of her life path, priests of our spiritual community gathered to meditate for several weeks on the name that would carry the vibration of her purpose. I was instructed that as a parent, I could chant my daughter's name whenever I needed to correct her path. When a child goes awry or faces confusion, chanting her spiritual name will help restore her equilibrium and her soul. I was also advised not to share her full name with anyone outside her family and immediate circle, as the name held power.

The same is true of many spiritual initiation processes in which the initiate is given a name chosen by priests or community elders to activate and hold the energy of the new archetypal, psychological, and spiritual energies they have been born into.

This ancestral wisdom still holds weight today. How many of us remember responding with immediate attention when one of our caregivers called us by our full name?

I always knew my mom meant business when she used my full name, the utterance of the sound calling me to proper order even before I knew what I had done wrong. In the modern fairy tale "Rumpelstiltskin" and many others, knowing one's name offers access to gifts, favors, blessings, and even esoteric wisdom.

Who are you trying to become in this phase of your soul development? I invite you to offer a sacred name for this aspect of yourself that is coming into being. This name might carry ancestral meaning or invoke the spirit of a plant or animal ally, or it may simply be a name that feels good to whisper, speak, or shout (hello, vibration!). Flex your throat chakra by translating this name into a gesture, creative movement, symbol, or drawing.

PRACTICE

ENERGIZE YOUR WATER

Here you can use the power of your voice to support your healing and transformation. Our bodies are more than 75 percent water, and the work of Masaru Emoto demonstrates that water molecules respond to negative and positive expressions.[9] They appear harmonious and orderly in response to life-supporting affirmations but are muddled

---

9   Masaru Emoto, *The Hidden Messages in Water* (Atria Books, 2005).

and disordered in reaction to negativity. Though Emoto's research methods have been deemed "unscientific" in some Western medical circles, his findings bring to light many Afro-Indigenous understandings of the nature of a vibrational universe. His experiments have sparked a larger conversation about the power of our thoughts and intentions.

Call to mind your intention and the qualities you'd like to cultivate. Know that this exercise is more effective when you focus on what you want to become (internal change) over what you what to achieve or acquire (external change). Make sure your intention is focused on your own inner growth and development as opposed to wanting to influence the thoughts, actions, or behaviors of another person. Whisper your prayer, your intention, or your affirmation into a glass of clear water. Make sure your breath is close enough to ripple the surface with vibration. Then, to embody this intention, sip your water throughout the day or offer it to a favorite plant.

NATURE'S PURE NECTAR CHAKRA

Our throat chakra holds the power to help us communicate to and through the natural world. This way of communication cares little about syntax, grammar, dialects, accent, or even the language we're speaking. Rather, communicating with nature relies on the energetic vibrations moderated by the fifth chakra.

Those of us who are animal lovers may have already experienced how our furry friends respond not primarily to our words but to the vibration of our expression, the tone of our voice, and our physical gestures. This is also the primary communication style of babies, demonstrating that energetic communication is encoded in our DNA. We come into the world knowing how to express ourselves, announcing our arrival on earth with our first breath. Considering that many behavioral scientists currently agree that most human communication is nonverbal, we are constantly using our throat chakra to communicate—even, and especially, without words.

PRACTICE

PLANT POSTURES

When studying plant medicine, we learn that the form and gesture of a plant often speaks to its psychological intention and intelligence. The shape and orientation of each plant gives us deep insight into its medicinal gift, its intelligence, and its aspiration for humanity. By embodying the gestures and forms of plants, we can enter a somatic conversation with the soul of nature. Our fifth chakra facilitates this silent conversation.

This meditative, imaginal practice helps us learn from our nonverbal teachers in the natural world. Find a plant or animal in your environment and take a moment to ground yourself. Feel your feet as they root down, experiencing the ground beneath you as the shared ancestor of humans, plants, and animals alike. As you hold the plant or animal in your attentive awareness, use your body to imitate the physical expression of the being. Do you raise your arms like branches to the sun? Do you tilt your head, just so, to mimic the graceful downward swoop of leaves? Perhaps balancing on one leg brings you deeper into shared form. Close your eyes to access wells of creativity as your throat chakra opens to this form of nonverbal expression. Journal, sketch, or sing any awareness that emerges from the form and gesture of your embodied somatic wisdom.

PRACTICE

ACUPRESSURE FOR DYNAMIC ENERGY PORTALS

In chapter 1, you learned about the meridians and nadis that carry energy throughout our bodies. In your mind's eye, picture these energetic rivers flowing from the top of your head to the bottoms of your feet. They traverse oceanic swells of energy centers, including the chakras. Each channel has dynamic energy portals, like mailboxes along a winding road that we use to communicate with the subtle body.

To engage the acupressure points below, rest your fingertips lightly on each as you look for a subtle sense of warmth or radiance. Use a light touch; your skin should not indent under your fingertips. You can also use vibrational remedies such as tuning forks, essential oils, flower essences, and gemstones on these points. See chapters 9 and 10 for vibrational remedies that resonate with the fifth chakra.

Conception Vessel 22: Tianshu (Celestial Chimney)

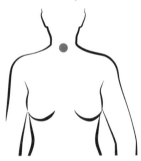

LOCATION: *On the midline at the base of the throat, in the bony depression at the top of the breastbone. Caution: use only light touch and gentle pressure on this point.*

In classical acupuncture theory, you can use the Window of Heaven points to activate the unique functions of CV22, or the Celestial Chimney point. These points are used to balance the connection between the heavenly and earthly aspects of the body and the spirit. They open a person to their true nature, forming a connection between the head and the rest of the body. This is an embodied way of experiencing the throat chakra as the bridge between the invisible (mind, ideas, and intention) and the visible world we create through our expression. Located at the base of the throat chakra, Tianshu is a point that helps strengthen and clarify the voice while opening the Window to Heaven to imbue our creative expression with inspiration.

Liver 3: Taichong (Supreme Surging)

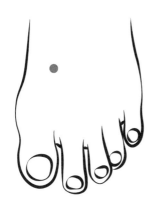

LOCATION: *Top of the foot, in the depression in the space between the metatarsal bones of your big toe and second toe.*

The liver meridian in traditional Chinese medicine is also very aligned with the throat chakra. It is used to address a lack of the confidence, clarity, and vision that are required for decisive action. It can be stimulated to either increase the volume or vitality of your voice or to soften a voice that is abrasive or condescending.

VISHUDDHA MUDRA VARIATION: BECOME THE HUM

This exercise can be grounding and regulatory, as it uses sound frequency to create resonance and equilibrium. The bija of the fifth chakra is *Ham* (pronounced "hum"). Each time you become the hum, you may discover a new sacred sound.

Begin by sitting in a comfortable place, with support for your lower back as needed. Gently roll your shoulders back and down as you lift the top of your head to the sky, allowing your neck to elongate. Turn your head from side to side and up and down to warm up your muscles and activate the Window to Heaven acupressure points that encircle the neck.

Now create the vishuddha mudra by interlacing your fingers on the inside of your hands (see illustration). Place the palms up, cradling your fingers as you press the tips of your thumbs together.

Call to mind a situation that requires your authentic voice or creative expression. Inhale deeply to fill your belly with spaciousness. On your exhale, press your lips together and allow a deep hum to emerge from your center. Sense

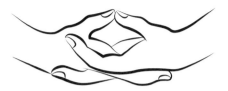

THE VISHUDDHA MUDRA

the vibration of the sound as it reverberates through your belly, throat, and lips. Repeat several times, experimenting with different tones, volumes, intensities, and pitches of sound until you find one that feels alive and resonant. Trust your body for an inner felt sense of "Yes!" or "That's it!"

Once you find this tone, repeat it until you feel a sense of balance and ease. Notice how your entire inner and outer being may be buzzing as you become the hum.

SUMMARY

The fifth chakra is a powerful portal to sounds of all sorts, which is why you can use words and names to stimulate, ease, and balance it. Use the acupuncture points shared in this chapter to enhance your work. Have fun trying these different exercises and compare how you communicate before and after.

7

SELF-HEALING AND GROUNDING

AMELIA VOGLER

In this chapter, you will deepen the healing potential of your fifth chakra and expand your ability to speak your authentic truth. You will gain new perspective on your throat chakra and learn practices to help open and balance this chakra, empowering you to share your truth and engage in authentic, honest conversations and interactions.

Meeting the world honestly is one of the most generative and healing energy exchanges the soul experiences. Consider how it feels to share your deepest desires, dreams, feelings, and experiences in a safe and supportive environment. These expressions become opportunities to be seen, heard, and acknowledged, and they may become cornerstone soul lessons. The ability to speak your truth opens a doorway to profound and lasting healing.

You cannot be fully in the world without sharing your truth. Unless you discover your voice and share it, a part of you will always be in hiding. It is a soul imperative that your truth, wisdom, and experience be added to the larger fields around you—those of your community, your family, your culture—and the ever-evolving universal field.

FOUNDATIONS FOR SELF-HEALING

To support your fifth chakra healing, I'd like to offer this foundational perspective: How and when you voice a message matters profoundly.

Whether you exchange messages with a family member, a client, a friend, or even yourself, you are responsible for any intuitive or subtle information you receive. Remember, energy is symbolic and metaphorical. Consider receiving the message "You are too sensitive." Literally, you might hear "There's something wrong with me." Energetically the message is "You express yourself in ways that are unique to you, and the speaker can't meet you in the fullness of who you really are."

Responsibility for expression also requires intentional timing. If you offer a transformative message or perspective when the listener is not ready, the message will never be received. If you offer it when someone is feeling disempowered, you risk their absorbing your message without the ability to discern whether it feels true for them.

Your pure nectar chakra is a vehicle of great power, and keeping these perspectives in your awareness is very important, even during quiet inner conversations with yourself.

PRACTICE

SOUNDING YOUR NAME: GROUNDING WHOLENESS

In this practice you will invoke your unique vibration by sounding your name. Your name's vibration is a collection of sounds, stories, inheritances, and ancestries. Chanting your name allows all you have been, all you are, and all you are becoming to flow through the fifth chakra and ground in your auric field. In essence, you are sounding yourself into wholeness.

Preparation

Your birth name holds a unique energy and story, just as your married, partnered, spiritual, or self-given names have their own. Decide which name to use for this practice.

Because this technique is about bringing your name as a mantra through your throat chakra, if you feel that parts of your name should be omitted due to strained relationships or histories, use the name or part of your name that feels most generative, alive, and loving. Consider chanting a self-given name or a nickname that resonates with you as another option.

Intention

To use your throat chakra to sound or chant your name as a personal mantra of wholeness and homecoming.

Steps

» Center yourself by taking a few deep, cleansing breaths.

» Feel, sense, and experience your body's boundary as a chamber.

» Practice sounding your name aloud. Try to hear it as simply sound and vibration.

» Once you have a sense of the vibration, with your eyes open, begin to chant your name.

» When the sound and vibration find a natural rhythm, close your eyes and continue to chant. Allow the vibration to fill the chamber of your body for as long as it feels supportive. Experiment with sounding your name at different speeds or pitches.

» Keeping your eyes closed, chant your name more and more quietly until there is silence. Allow the vibration to continue into the silence

> the way the sound of a gong slowly disappears
> but the feeling of the sound continues to ring.

You have become your own tuning fork, harmonizing your vibration with your body and the world beyond.

PRACTICE

SPEAKING YOUR BOUNDARIES

There are a few words that, when spoken, instantly assert your boundaries: "yes," "no," and "not right now." Consider how often you think about these boundaries rather than vocalizing them. Most often we do boundary work in the privacy of our inner world, and only when boundaries are most needed do we speak them aloud.

This practice encourages you to freely speak your boundaries aloud, even in solitude. Your literal and energetic boundaries are clarified and strengthened when you allow voice and intention to marry in vocalization. This simple practice is a healing tonic for the throat chakra, enabling it to open and flow with the energies of your truth. The practice also creates energetic templates for expressing boundaries: well-traveled pathways that flow from your throat chakra and make speaking your boundaries more accessible. When you develop these templates, it becomes easier to live honestly with yourself.

Preparation

Consider a situation in which you wish to clarify or strengthen your boundaries. This can be in any area of your life: work, friendships, family, or even a conflict you are struggling with internally. Give yourself as much time as you need to think about and explore the tender edges of your boundaries. Remember, you have an inner boundary and an outer one. The inner one helps you manage safe and healthy energies to share with the world; ask yourself what you are willing to share with another person or an experience. The outer boundary keeps you protected from external energies that don't serve you; ask yourself what is no longer healthy or tolerable.

Grab a pen and paper for this practice.

Intention

To allow the vibrations of the words "yes," "no," and "not right now" to imprint boundaries in your energy field.

Steps

> » Call to mind a struggle or situation for which you wish to imprint boundaries.

> » Classify aspects of this situation by writing down what you say "no," "yes," and "not right now" to. Grouping what you say into these classifications will generate lists of boundaries.

Work with these until they are complete, clear, and well stated.

» Speak aloud each boundary in your "no" list. You will release affirmations of this boundary through your energy field as you do this. Feel, sense, or experience your "no" boundary becoming clear and sturdy.

» Speak aloud each boundary in your "not right now" list. Feel, sense, or experience the protection and support of these positive boundaries as they give you more time and space.

» Speak aloud each boundary in your "yes" list. Feel, sense, or experience your energy allowing relationship and the exchange of energy.

» Process how you feel, and note any questions. Repeat these steps as needed.

This practice does not require that you know how to enact these boundaries. Some actions may come easily and naturally, while at other times right action comes later, after some thought. Be patient, and seek support as needed.

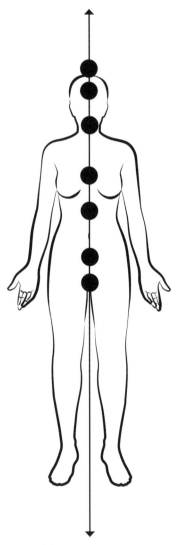

THE HARA LINE

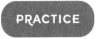

ACCESSING THE VOICE OF YOUR SOUL

When the throat chakra is fully expanded, it radiates and channels energies received from the hands (consider the messages received from automatic writing) and the ears (consider auditory messages). These are ways you express truth, but from where does your voice originate? The voice of your authentic self, or your soul, resides in your hara dimension.

The hara line is a vertical energy dimension that manages the design and flow of your incarnation. It organizes your authentic spiritual codes, your soul's incarnation purpose, your relationship to your body, and even your relationship to the planet. When performing optimally, it bonds you to heaven and grounds you to the earth.

This dimension primarily flows through the center of your being. It creates a central channel of energy, guiding its flow from the point of your soul's individuation from the universal field down to the core of the earth and back up. The hara energy flows up and down the center line, which in the physical body incorporates your spine. You can see it on page 122.

The hara energy carries the unique, authentic energy codes of your soul, particularly the codes required for an upcoming incarnation. The codes for this life might be slightly different than those related to an earlier life, but that is because your soul has different tasks to embody. The hara energy brings your soul's essence and wisdom into all your energy systems; these include the chakras, nadis, meridians, and the dantians, which are energy centers in many forms of traditional Chinese medicine that are rooted in Taoist and Buddhist philosophies.

In the chakra system, the very center of each chakra connects to the hara line, which in turn relates to your essence. This innermost chakra energy holds your truth, and the hara energy sources the energy templates within each chakra to be activated and empowered.

When accessing the energy of your authentic voice and its inner messages, you must practice grounding your hara. This will allow you to both connect with and express your truth.

Preparation

Find a quiet, comfortable space for this exercise. Bring paper and pen if you like to journal or process through writing. If you love color or art, gather paper and colored pencils. Bring your personal practices to your tool kit too, such as deep breathing and mindful focus, to steady and clear your mind of chatter. If you have a naturally chatty mind, try extending your exhalation longer than your inhalation for a few cycles as you begin this practice.

Coming to this practice well-grounded in your chakras allows the chakras to stay open and receptive to expressing the energy of your soul. If needed, perform a simple grounding exercise: Visualize yourself as a tree with your roots deep in the ground. Feel or imagine Mother Earth's energy flowing upward through all seven main chakras, beginning with the first (at the base of your coccyx) and ending at the crown (at the top of the head). Take all the time you need to feel your chakras open and flowing. Consider spending a little more time at the throat chakra or employ some of the other techniques offered in this chapter to help engage this chakra's energy frequency.

Intention

To access the voice of your soul by accessing your hara dimension.

Steps

» Either seated in a chair or standing, maintain a straight spine. Feel your feet on the ground or floor beneath you or connect with the ground through intention.

» Close your eyes or soften your gaze.

» Allow your hands to rest comfortably in your lap, or, if standing, let them rest palms open in front of you.

» Visualize, feel, or imagine the earth below your feet and the celestial universe above you.

» Intentionally connect to the star that has your name on it—the one star that carries your soul energy in this lifetime.

» Visualize, feel, or imagine a stream of light from that star flowing down through your crown, down your central channel, and out through your perineum, running down past the earth's surface, past the underground riverways, past the lava fields, all the way down to the center of Mother Earth, into her radiant ball of crystalline light at the center.

» Allow your energy to blend and merge with her crystalline core. In this way, reunite with your first mother, who supports your life in all ways.

» By intention, bring this blended energy back up through the layers of the earth, through the perineum, up the central channel, back out through the crown of your head, and upward to the star with your name on it.

- » Feel these downward and upward flows of energy in your central channel. This is your hara energy.

- » Bring your awareness to your throat and ask, "What message does my soul bring to me?"

- » Allow the answer to come through written words, drawings, or auditory messages.

- » Ground yourself by tapping or stomping your feet on the ground and bringing movement and intentional breath to the body.

- » From this grounded place, look for the symbols, metaphors, and patterns in your message. Consider their meaning in your life.

SUMMARY

The fifth chakra is the portal to speaking your truth, whether expressing the guiding messages of your authentic self, enacting your internal and external boundaries, or calling forth your wholeness through vibration. Consider the throat chakra as a vehicle for the right relationship with yourself, the most authentic expression of your honesty and integrity. The practices in this chapter will build the scaffolding needed to know yourself and speak your truth.

8

GUIDED MEDITATIONS

AMANDA HUGGINS

The fifth chakra is connected to the energy of communication, expression, and the ability to speak one's truth. Although meditation is often a silent practice, it is still a powerful tool for aligning and activating the energy of communication and expression.

Meditation techniques such as focused breathing and visualization can help release blockages in the fifth chakra, thus allowing the energy to circulate freely. In the quietude of meditation, you can attune yourself to your inner voice, gain insights into your authentic thoughts and feelings, and increase trust in your ability to express yourself honestly, openly, and from a place of truth.

Some meditation practices go beyond silent contemplation and actively encourage you to use your voice. In mantra meditations, you're invited to repeat or chant a specific sound or word, creating a rhythmic resonance that aligns with the vibrational frequencies of an energy center. Whether you choose to remain silent or use your voice in meditation focused on the throat chakra, these practices facilitate the expression of genuine emotions and ideas when engaging with others.

While the fifth chakra is most often associated with the throat, its influence extends far beyond just the throat space and vocal expression. This energy center also involves the ears—specifically, your capacity to hear and receive balanced communication from others. It also encompasses your ability to receive information from beyond the physical realm, such as intuitive hits or clairaudient guidance.

Meditation can facilitate both articulate speech and a profound ability to hear, fostering deeper connections with others and an openness to the wisdom of Spirit. Through regular practice, you can deeply activate the energy of the throat chakra and develop the ability to communicate with compassion and empathy.

MEDITATING AND CONNECTING WITH THE THROAT CHAKRA

In this chapter, you will experience three different throat chakra meditations, each offering a slightly different access point for connecting with and activating the throat chakra.

In the first meditation, you'll use the power of color-based visualization to connect with, clear, and charge your throat chakra. In the second meditation, you'll harmonize your vocal energy through audible repetition of a statement that aligns with the throat chakra. The third meditation is a creative visualization. You'll be guided on a dynamic visual journey that empowers you to express your throat chakra and unlock the full potential of your voice.

For all meditations focused on this energy center, a suitable meditative posture is a comfortable seated position. The spine should be erect and aligned, promoting alertness and receptivity. An upright position encourages an open and expansive chest, allowing breath to flow freely. This openness extends to the throat and will create a clear pathway for the energy and vibration of the fifth chakra to move through your physical and subtle bodies.

PRACTICE

COLOR-BASED VISUALIZATION FOR THROAT CHAKRA HEALING

There are no real requirements for this meditation; however, if you'd like to support your mind and energy in connecting more deeply, you might consider lighting a blue candle or gently holding a blue crystal in your hand. (Crystals like aquamarine, lapis lazuli, blue kyanite, or blue calcite are my personal favorites.)

To begin, find a comfortable seat in a quiet space where you won't be disturbed. Gently close your eyes and begin to breathe deeply.

Scan the body for any areas that are holding resistance, and use your exhales to softly release any tension. Pay particular attention to the shoulder, jaw, and throat area. Unclench the jaw and swallow a few times to release any tension in the throat. You may repeat this practice of scanning and releasing until the entire throat chakra region feels soft and unrestricted. Allow the breath to find a natural, relaxed rhythm.

Rest your awareness in the true center of your throat and visualize a radiant blue light swirling there in a counterclockwise motion. As you place more attention in this area, you may notice a slight tingling or tapping sensation in the throat. If you get the urge to clear your throat, don't resist it: simply clear it and return to the breath.

Continue focusing on this radiant ball of blue energy. Observe the size, shape, vibrancy, and texture of this chakra without judgment. You may also note the speed and intensity of the light. Remember that there is no "wrong" way to visualize; this is a practice in working with your intuitive guidance.

With each breath, allow yourself to intuitively adjust the blue light. You may choose to play with brightness, speed, size, or vibration. As you play with your adjustments, ask yourself what feels most comfortable for you today. For example, perhaps your light first appeared as a dull blue and it would feel better for you to increase the intensity. Or perhaps the light was vibrating at a speed that felt uncomfortably fast for you and you'd like to turn it down. Again, there is no "wrong" way to adjust; you're just tuning your personal dials.

When you feel your chakra has been adequately adjusted, allow that blue light to expand from the center of the throat. With each breath, see it enveloping the entire body. Witness how far the light travels and just receive the energy. Continue to breathe deeply. Use your exhales to release any tension or emotional resistance that come up, and use your inhales to replenish those emptied spaces with the felt sensation of authenticity. Allow yourself to take up as much space as you can.

Continue breathing in this beautiful aura of blue light for as long as you'd like, savoring any positive sensations you're experiencing.

When you're ready to conclude, gently draw that aura of beautiful blue light back into your throat chakra.

Shift your awareness back to your breath's cadence. Deepen your breath, gradually bringing more energy into your body and the space around you. When you feel ready, open your eyes and return to your surroundings.

PRACTICE

MANTRA MEDITATION FOR VIBRATIONAL RESONANCE

This meditation will have you engaging in a simple affirmation: "I am powerfully expressing." This affirmation captures the essence of fifth chakra energy, emphasizing the qualities of genuine and honest self-expression. When repeated with intention and focus, this mantra can help align and balance the energy of the throat chakra, fostering clear communication and authenticity in your daily life interactions.

When you're ready to begin, find a comfortable seated position. Bring your hands together and interlock the pinky, ring, and middle fingers, bending them over the tops of your hands. From that interlock, connect the tips of the thumbs with the index fingers to form two rings, almost as if you were making the "okay" hand signal with both hands. This is the Granthita mudra, a symbolic gesture associated with the energy of the throat chakra.

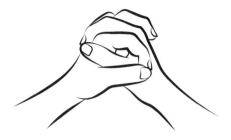

THE GRANTHITA MUDRA

Close the eyes gently and take a few deep breaths to settle into the present moment. Allow your breath to arrive at a natural, melodic rhythm.

Shift your attention to the throat area. Notice and feel the gentle rise and fall of your breath in this region.

As you inhale, repeat aloud: "I am . . ."

As you exhale, repeat aloud: "powerfully expressing."

Continue repeating this affirmation, syncing your words with the rise and fall of your breath.

Feel the resonance of this affirmation in your throat chakra. Play with the volume, pitch, tone, and length of your words. Eventually, you will find the frequency of "I am powerfully expressing" that feels right in your throat and your voice. Feel the resonance of these words in your throat and allow it to reverberate through your being, cleansing and aligning the throat chakra.

Let yourself get lost in the sound and vibration of "I am powerfully expressing." As you immerse yourself in this mantra, it will become a rhythmic gateway into a deeper meditative state. The simple, continuous repetition will also help prevent the mind from wandering into distractions, allowing you to enter a deep state of awareness and presence.

Continue this meditation for a few more minutes, maintaining a focused and intentional connection with your words. With each repetition, sense the mantra deepening its impact on the throat chakra, clearing out any old energy and creating more space for your authentic voice.

When you feel complete with your chanting, sit in silence for a minute. Notice how the mantra's resonance lingers in your awareness.

To close the meditation, deepen the breath. Gently open your eyes and bring your awareness back to the present moment.

PRACTICE

GUIDED VISUALIZATION:
SEE YOURSELF USING YOUR VOICE

This guided visualization serves as a safe space to visualize using your voice and engaging in clear, empathic, and expressive communication. As you hone your ability to articulate and express in the meditative realm, you'll cultivate the confidence to carry those skills into the real world. Visualization serves as a transformative process, where the scenes you create in meditation begin to integrate into your daily interactions, enhancing your communications with clarity, sincerity, and a profound ability to connect to your true voice.

Begin in a quiet space and find a comfortable seat. Spend a few minutes relaxing the entire body. Connect with the natural rhythm of your breath.

Imagine yourself in a serene, fully white space, a calming blank canvas upon which you'll create a scene to explore your ideal self-expression.

Identify the desires of your throat chakra. For example, do you wish you could be more expressive in your day-to-day life? Or perhaps you'd like to use your voice to better protect your energy through boundary-setting or clear communication. On the other hand, you may have a desire to develop better listening or empathic communication skills. There is no "wrong" answer; simply tune in to the center of your throat chakra and feel for what is most needed.

With that answer in mind, create a visual scene in your mind's eye. Let this scene fulfill the desires of the fifth chakra. If you wish for more expressiveness, envision your-self confidently communicating your thoughts and feelings with authenticity. If your desire relates to setting boundar-ies, visualize yourself calmly and assertively communicat-ing your needs. If you desire improved listening or empa-thetic communication skills, imagine a scenario where you are fully present in a conversation with a loved one.

When you've clarified your visualization, wrap the entire mental scene in a soft blue light and watch the scene play out to your highest and best good. As you do, engage all your senses. Feel the resonance in your throat as you speak and listen. Experience the feelings of joy, clarity, and authenticity in your body. Feel the expansive power of your throat chakra activating in real-life scenarios.

You may choose to replay the scene a few times, each round focusing more intently on creating real feelings and sensations in your body. Spend a few moments softly dwell-ing in your visualized reality, allowing the positive energy of your fulfilled desires to resonate throughout the physical and energetic body.

When you feel complete with the visualization, allow the mental scene to fade. Draw your awareness back to your breath and your body, then gently open the eyes.

As you move about your day, see if you can maintain the positive feelings you elicited in this meditation.

SUMMARY

Meditation in all forms—silent or audible—is a wonderful practice that can enhance harmonious connection between your conscious self and the energy of your fifth chakra. Through mindful techniques such as color visualization, mantra repetition, and creative visualization, you'll create pathways to unlock the transformative power of the throat chakra and foster clarity, confidence, and a profound alignment with your true voice.

9

VIBRATIONAL REMEDIES

JO-ANNE BROWN

In the late 1960s, seventy monks lived at Abbaye d'En Cal-cat, a monastery in Southern France. Many of them slept only four to six hours per night, but they were healthy, hardworking, and emotionally balanced. When they suddenly became fatigued and depressed, health professionals from near and far were consulted, but none of their recommended solutions made a difference.

An ear specialist named Alfred Tomatis was then called upon to help. He discovered that the newly appointed abbot had ended the monks' daily practice of chanting as they worked, believing it served no purpose. After receiving a practitioner-led vibrational remedy and after chanting was restored as a normal part of their daily routine, the monks' good health returned.[10]

10 Norman Doidge, MD, *The Brain's Way of Healing: Remarkable Discoveries and Recoveries from the Frontiers of Neuroplasticity* (Penguin Life, 2016), 343.

This experience confirmed what Tomatis believed: that certain types of music are rich in high-frequency harmonics. By hearing their own voices expressing their spiritual truths through chanting, the monks were activating their pure nectar chakra. They were also benefiting from a secondary function of hearing: recharging their brain and nervous system energy.[11]

This inspirational true story is my favorite example of the healing power of fifth chakra vibrational remedies.

In this chapter, I share my understanding of these vibrational remedies and

> » explain what they are

> » describe their benefits

> » share my preferred practice-based and tangible fifth chakra remedies

> » outline two practices to help you support your fifth chakra at home

WHAT ARE VIBRATIONAL REMEDIES?

Vibrational remedies are practices and medicines of a vibrational nature that create and allow for natural balance and flow.

11 Jonathan Goldman, *Healing Sounds: The Power of Harmonics* (Healing Arts Press, 2002), 120–22.

When healthy expression is not enabled in our throat chakra, we are not sharing our core signature vibration. We may be reticent to speak our truth and share our creative expression or, alternatively, we may express ourselves in a dominating way.

When we experience vibrational remedies created specifically for our pure nectar chakra, we can more easily hear and express our personal truths in our daily lives.

WHAT IS RESONANCE?

Resonance is a natural phenomenon that occurs when an object vibrating at its preferred frequency reaches optimal strength, or amplitude.

Bone conduction is a form of resonance specific to the fifth chakra. It differs from air conduction because the vibrational sound is transmitted directly to the bones of the skull rather than through the medium of air. In turn, the sounds are transmitted to the internal ear components embedded in the temporal skull bone, and resonance with the cranial (skull) bones allows the sound vibration to strengthen.

When we experience specially crafted remedies that support our personal truth, like the monks in France, we too are activating our pure nectar chakra.

THE YIN AND YANG OF
OUR PURE NECTAR CHAKRA

The dual concept of yin and yang is fundamental to the practice of traditional Chinese medicine (TCM). Each represents a polar opposite of the duality, where yin is receptive and yang is expressive.

Within our fifth chakra, our ears represent the yin/receptive aspect, while our vocal workings represent the yang/outwardly expressive aspect.

Researchers have discovered that the voice produces only what the ear hears and the brain processes.[12] This discovery reflects the functioning of our internal auditory feedback loop (AFL), a three-part cyclical process where (1) we speak, (2) we hear and listen to what we have said, and (3) we cognitively process what we have verbally expressed. The third step is crucial: It allows us to make corrections where necessary so our words reflect our personal truth. When our internal AFL is working well, we communicate easily and effectively.

By extension, if we can't hear or receive our spiritual truths, we are literally unable to understand our truths cognitively or verbally express them.

---

12 Tomatis Australia, "What Is the Tomatis Method?" https://tomatis.com
.au/what-is-the-tomatis-method/.

Sound and frequency experts are aware that certain types of music contain all the frequencies of the voice spectrum, which fall between 70 Hz and 9,000 Hz. When we haven't been exposed to this full frequency range, vibrational remedies are able to fill in the gaps physically, psychologically, and spiritually.[13]

VIBRATIONAL REMEDIES FOR YOUR FIFTH CHAKRA

Vibrational remedies fall into one of two categories:

- » practice-based
- » tangible

Practice-Based Vibrational Remedies

Practice-based remedies include subtle energy treatments, therapies, and practices that require the guidance of a qualified practitioner. They support our pure nectar chakra energies through:

- » direct skin contact, including acupuncture and massage
- » vibrational media, including sound therapies and frequency-based modalities
- » demonstrational guidance, including yoga

---

13 Jonathan Goldman, *Healing Sounds: The Power of Harmonics* (Healing Arts Press, 2002), 122.

Based on my experience, the most effective practice-based remedies for the throat chakra are sound-based, so I will highlight three such therapies that are beneficial for throat chakra support.

FREQUENCY-BASED MODALITIES. Frequency-generating instruments, such as the Rife machine, are used to intentionally send therapeutic vibrations into the body through conductive electrodes. The most supportive vibrations for the fifth chakra's associated organs can stimulate sympathetic resonance, which means that these healthy vibrations cause other areas to move at the same frequencies. In traditional Chinese medicine, this balancing occurs within related organs and meridians. This supports core bodily systems and counteracts degenerative disease patterns, resulting in improved health.

Of the TCM meridians, the Triple Warmer meridian is most closely aligned with the fifth chakra due to its association with the thyroid gland.

When the Triple Warmer meridian is stimulated using 10 Hz and 30 kHz, fifth chakra energetic blockages can be released. Thyroid blockages can also be reduced with 6.4 Hz and

128 kHz, and blockages in the cervical vertebrae can be released with 7.4 Hz and 127 kHz.

For the fifth chakra, I also recommend the use of solfeggio tuning forks to access healing solfeggio frequencies, especially 528 Hz, one of three solfeggio frequencies that relate to numerology's soul or spiritual plane. The other two are 285 Hz and 852 Hz.

AUDITORY FEEDBACK MODALITIES. These modalities employ the use of auditory feedback devices to improve sensory processing, sound discrimination, voice quality, and reading ability. The best-known practitioner-led modality of this kind uses a device called the Electronic Ear and is called the Tomatis Method, created by the ear specialist who helped the ailing monks in France.

There are also home-based auditory feedback devices that do not require a trained practitioner.

Upon registering a speech sample, these devices modulate the sample by making specific frequencies louder (as a fully functioning ear would do). The altered vocal sounds are received by the ears, allowing the auditory feedback loop to be retrained.

I have personally experienced a number of these devices and prefer the Forbrain headset device since it is a highly effective and easily accessible option.

SOUND THERAPY: EXPOSURE TO HIGH-FREQUENCY HARMONIC MUSIC. In general, classical music heightens our emotional state, enabling us to be more receptive to learning. More specifically, research has identified that Gregorian chants and music composed by Mozart, particularly his violin concertos, contain high-frequency harmonics of about 8,000 Hz. By listening to such music, our auditory feedback loop is activated, improving concentration and neurological patterning in the brain cortex.

Tangible Vibrational Remedies

These remedies are physical solutions that correct fifth chakra imbalances.

The most common physical remedies include a carrier such as water, a preserving agent such as alcohol, and the vibrational remedy itself.

These remedies are particularly appropriate for the throat chakra as many of them are ingestible by mouth or under the tongue before being absorbed into the bloodstream.

HOMEOPATHIC REMEDIES. Homeopathy is an alternative medicine that treats dysfunction and dis-ease using minute doses of natural substances, including plants and minerals, that would ordinarily produce the same dysfunction and dis-ease in larger doses.

A qualified homeopathy practitioner will prescribe remedies at a suitable resonating potency to produce a curative reaction in the patient without disturbing or damaging the body.

Homeopathic remedies that promote healthy fifth chakra energies include Kali iodatum (for colds and cough discharges), Fucus vesiculosus (for thyroid conditions), Carcinosin (for ear disorders), Acidum salicylicum (for diminished hearing, tinnitus, and tonsillitis), and Apis mellifica (for ear infections).

FLOWER ESSENCES. These remedies have been used for centuries to support and balance the human body and mind. Unlike essential oils, they are received into the mouth in droplet form, preferably under the tongue. Those I list here have fifth chakra qualities and benefits I've personally experienced or observed in my clients.

» *Bach flower remedies:* Among the thirty-eight remedies in this range of essences created by Dr. Edward Bach, I recommend two for the throat chakra: Agrimony (for authentic communication) and Holly (for generous self-expression).

» *Elementals flower essence range:* These essences were created by Lindsay Fauntleroy, medicine maker, educator, and author of chapter 6 of this book. My two favorites for the fifth chakra are Eloquence (for clear communication and creative expression) and Queendom (for intuitive listening and genuine sharing).

» *Australian bushflower essences:* As an Australian-based healer, I've worked with this extensive flower essence range, created by Australian herbalist Ian White, for decades. My preferred remedies for the fifth chakra include Creative Essence (for healthy self-expression), Relationship Essence (for enhanced communication), Bush Fuchsia (for courage to share your truth), Five Corners (for enhanced self-expression), and Flannel Flower (for difficulty in communicating feelings).

Following are two vibrational practices to support your throat chakra.

IMPROVE YOUR PURE NECTAR CHAKRA INTUITION

This practice can be enjoyed as a single experience or be added to your daily routine for more profound benefits.

- » Choose a time of day when you can spend thirty minutes undisturbed.

- » Select one or more pieces of music that contain high-frequency harmonics, such as music composed by Mozart (especially violin concertos) or Gregorian chants.

- » Make yourself comfortable, relax, and play your chosen music for thirty minutes. Ensure that the speaker is close to your left ear, which is more sensitive to registering emotions, intuition, and music.

- » After each session, observe and reflect on how you are feeling. Record your observations in a dedicated notebook. If you are using this as a daily practice, be aware of any changes in your emotional and intuitive receptivity over time.

Note: This practice can be adapted to support improved speech and logic in the following ways:

» Put the speaker close to your right ear
instead; this allows the sound to reach the
speech centers in your brain more quickly
and improves your focus, memory retention,
listening abilities, and educational performance.

» Throughout your listening or right afterward,
observe and reflect on your mental clarity and
be aware of any changes in your ability to focus
and retain knowledge.

PRACTICE

ENHANCE YOUR ABILITY TO
COMMUNICATE AUTHENTICALLY

Prior to commencing this practice, you may wish to take
some flower essence drops or a homeopathic remedy recommended earlier in this chapter that supports your self-
expression and allows clear communication.

» Find a place where you can do this practice
without interruptions.

» Place your right hand gently on your throat
and say these words: "I speak my own truth
in all situations." Continue to repeat these
words and get a sense of how true they are
to you in the here and now. Check to see if
you are feeling a rising, buoyant sensation in

your throat or a sinking sensation. If you are feeling an optimistic, rising energy, you are resonating with your words and they are your truth. If your energy feels like it is sinking and bottoming out, you are not resonating with your words and they are not your truth.

» Consider how you can change your words so you are speaking your truth. A more truthful statement for you at this time may be "I am learning to speak my own truth in all situations." Again, check for rising or sinking energy in your throat to determine whether you are speaking your truth or not.

» Continue to revise your statements until you come to a place where you know you are speaking your truth. Continuing this theme, you may check for internal resonance with the following statements:

> *I speak my own truth when it*
> *doesn't hurt the feelings of others.*

> *I speak my own truth when*
> *I feel strong and well balanced.*

> *I choose my words carefully so*
> *I can more easily speak my own truth.*

» As you do this practice, recognize that you are strengthening your internal auditory feedback loop and your ability to discern and correct your words and speak your genuine truth.

SUMMARY

When we work with vibrational remedies that support the pure nectar chakra, we are reminded of our own inherent truth and are encouraged to express that in the world. In this chapter you learned about remedies and practices that facilitate this expression and support all aspects of your receptive, discerning, and expressive fifth chakra.

10

CRYSTALS, MINERALS, AND STONES

MARGARET ANN LEMBO

Using gemstones to focus on calibrating your fifth chakra is a powerful way to shape up your communication skills physically, mentally, emotionally, and spiritually. Basically, you can choose varying shades of light blue and turquoise gemstones to rebalance and align your throat center.

The main colors of the fifth chakra are sky blue and turquoise; other shades of blue can be used as well. Enhancing the vibration of blue at the throat using various crystals and gemstones can bring about feelings of peace, ease in communication, and connection with messages from the Divine, invisible celestial helpers, spiritual guides, and those who have passed over. Aided by fifth chakra stones, you can make these contacts easily and safely.

Benefiting this energy center will always help you express yourself and listen to others. Following are areas in which gemstones can aid your throat chakra.

COMMUNICATION VIA THE FIFTH CHAKRA

Your fifth chakra is essentially about communication, which includes speaking, expressing, and listening, as well as truly hearing what someone is sharing with you. We may tend to think about something else while someone is speaking or respond before truly hearing them. Being grounded and present in the moment is an important factor in being a good listener, and there are gemstones that can help.

DIVINE TIMING

The throat chakra is the place to focus when you want to connect with and receive guidance from spirit guides and angels. These heavenly beings can co-orchestrate your life, assuring that you are always in the right place at the right time with the right people. Some experiences may seem like coincidences, but when you are connected with divine alignment, events that seem synchronistic are often a result of divine timing. You can live a charmed life and allow for an easy flow when your intention is to be exactly where you are supposed to be.

WORD PATROL

Words create reality. What you say and think vibrates and comes right back to you. Every statement, thought, and word manifests your reality. Use self-observation and become aware of what you are drawing to you. Pay attention when thinking or saying things like "You are making me crazy" or "This is killing me"—then self-correct to create a healthier, more balanced life.

When a gemstone is paired with a verbal intention, the stone amplifies that intention and helps you maintain your focus on it. Focus on the image or thought of your intention and then look at the choices of crystals available to you, such as in a store or in your private collection. I'll be providing my recommendations on which stones to use. If you are attracted to a gemstone while choosing crystals, go with your gut and with what you find attractive. Match your positive thoughts with that gemstone and watch your world realign with what you want to create.

Following are amazing gemstones for activating your throat chakra and its potential.

Amazonite is the stone of truth and honesty. This blue-green stone helps you focus on your truth and improves your ability to be comfortable speaking and living your truth. If you tend to hold back something that needs to be said, grab a piece of amazonite and make your intention to speak up with grace, compassion, and love. Employ amazonite affirmations like these: *It's easy for me to say what is on my mind. I have the courage to speak up for myself and express my truth.*

Angelite is a good stone to use when you need to be a better listener. Sky blue, it carries the ability to sort out your thoughts, put them aside, and hear what others say. It's a great gem for opening yourself to receive guidance and messages from invisible helpers like angels and guides. Great affirmations for this stone include these: *I am a good listener. Guidance and messages from higher realms of consciousness help me daily.*

Aquamarine, a blue beryl, is great to have on hand to express watery emotions. Use it to maintain poise when you are expressing verbally or telepathically. This stone of truth brings compassion and tolerance for yourself and others when emotions are communicated. Clear away accumulated negative emotions to bring ease during unsettling conversations or internal dialogue. Try these affirmations or make up similar ones of your own: *I am emotionally balanced when I express my feelings. I am safe when I feel my feelings. I express myself with ease and grace.*

Blue calcite is extremely calming. It's lovely for when you need to chill out your anger and shift toward peaceful acceptance. It's also a perfect gem to improve how you communicate. This sky blue stone helps fill you with grace and diplomacy. Blue calcite is an excellent ally when writing your feelings in a journal or a letter. It helps make you more aware of how you express and employ "word patrol" when necessary. Here are some fantastic affirmations for accessing this stone's magic: *I am peaceful even when the world around me changes. I am compassionate with myself and others. I hear, see, and know messages from Spirit.*

Blue lace agate and blue chalcedony are related stones. Use either to improve your communication skills, including how well you hear and understand what others are expressing. They encourage calming vibrations and reduce inflamed emotions. Use these stones to help you recognize divine timing in your life. Employ affirmations like these: *I am peaceful and communicate with ease. I am a good listener. I am grateful that I am always where I need to be and with the right people.*

Turquoise is another gemstone that helps you know, speak, and live your truth. It's a great stone to help you tap into the Akashic Records—the recordings of all events across time—and communicate with the angels. Hold some turquoise and ask the angels to co-orchestrate your days so you can live your best life. These affirmations can help you do exactly that: *I am connected with the records of the universe. Insight and wisdom come to my awareness from various cultures and philosophies. I know my truth and live it daily.*

COMMUNICATION WITH ALL LIFE

As you develop spiritually, your conscious awareness expands and you recognize that you can communicate with plants, animals, birds, and all life. There are stones you can work with to improve interspecies communication. The fifth chakra stones listed below can be any color, shape, or size.

Andalusite is also known as chiastolite. This stone is ideal for communicating with the earth plane's devic forces and invisible realms. Carbonaceous inclusions form a black cross in this stone, adding to its grounding nature. Enjoy a deeper relationship with plants and trees with this stone in hand, and think about using these affirmations to do so: *The energies of nature are wise. I listen to the fairies and devic forces of the earth.*

Tabular clear quartz is beneficial to work with for telepathic communication. You can recognize it because two sides of the crystal are much wider than the other four, and it is flat and tablet-like. Try on these affirmations to create optimum communication: *I communicate from my heart to the hearts of animals and plants. It's easy to send mental pictures to express myself. I am aware of messages from nature.*

Brown agate is earthy brown and serves as a good tool for grounding your awareness as you connect with the earth. Hold a piece of it to tap into the elemental world of your houseplants, garden, and all nature. Use this stone to awaken and remember to communicate with all life. You are a steward of the earth and are responsible for how you care for the environment. The following affirmations are designed to optimize this stone: *It is easy for me to be a good caretaker of the earth. I have a green thumb because I listen to the plants in my home and garden.*

Larimar is a blue-green stone that looks like the ocean. It is ideal for telepathic communication with animals. Hold a piece of larimar to improve your animal communication skills. Breathe deeply, connect with your pets or with any animals, and you'll know what they need or want. Be open to receiving their messages in thoughts or pictures in your mind, employing affirmations like these to access larimar's powers: *I know and understand unspoken communication. Dogs, cats, birds, and all life commune with me, and I comprehend what they communicate.*

IMAGINING A GEMSTONE AROUND YOU

Imagine you are holding a light blue or turquoise gemstone; you can select any of the stones in this chapter and visualize its color. Then envision the shade of that gemstone turning into a bubble around you.

The bubble resonates with feelings of peace. There are angels and invisible helpers in this blue energy that watch over you and guide you. You feel protected and connected to the Divine, even as this colorful energy helps you feel comfortable saying what you need to express. It is your reminder that you can receive guidance from otherworldly beings like angels, spirit guides, and loved ones who have passed away.

PRACTICE

OPENING THE THROAT

Visualize a band of energy swirling around your neck that is the color of a gemstone you relate to. Use your imagination to tap into your communication skills, encompassing thoughts, feelings, pictures, and words. Feel the link between yourself and all life—humans, nature, animals, and beyond.

SUMMARY

A balanced throat chakra helps you communicate easily with everyone and all life. When the throat chakra is calibrated, you will know your personal truth and feel comfortable living your truth. You can use the gemstones described in this chapter to relate to all throat chakra capabilities and connect with spirit guides and angels to receive their messages and guidance. With the assistance of crystals and stones, you will see, hear, know, feel, smell, and taste truth on a metaphysical level—beyond the ordinary—and let life become easier.

11

MANTRA HEALING

BLAKE TEDDER

Devotional singing is a terrific practice for healing and activating the throat chakra. I love devotional singing of all kinds: Christian Taizé singing, Gregorian chants, Pakistani *qawwali*, Sufi *zikr*, pagan circle songs, and more. All bring the throat chakra into expression by interweaving sound with sacred words, themes, and feelings. I have been especially drawn to *kirtan*: call-and-response devotional singing of holy mantras from Hindu and Sikh religious traditions. Through my explorations in kirtan as a chant leader and kirtan radio show host, I have encountered many styles and flavors of devotional singing in both traditional and Western contexts. One thing is clear: Singing mantras is a fun and powerful practice for opening the throat chakra and for personal transformation.

WHAT IS A MANTRA?

Mantras are sacred or spiritual sounds, words, or phrases that are repeated, chanted, sung, or meditated upon for various purposes. Generally, they are especially effective at cleaning, repatterning, and tonifying our energy systems. There are thousands of mantras traditionally linked with Hindu deities, Buddhas, Tibetan historical figures, and Sikh gurus. They can be invoked for just about any spiritual or health-related purpose, almost always for healing and realization. The word *mantra* itself comes from the ancient Sanskrit language combining *manas,* or "the thinking mind," with *trā,* or "instrument/tool." These potent tools, when wielded with respect and expectation of their power, quickly create the conditions for major change.

MANTRAS, SANSKRIT, AND THE POWER OF SOUND

The Sanskrit language, which is the source of most mantras, is an ancient Indo-Aryan language with a rich tradition that is found in spiritual and religious texts, particularly in Hinduism, Buddhism, and Jainism. It is a dynamic language renowned for its phonetic precision, where the sounds carry unique vibrations, rendering mantras spiritually potent. Its complex grammatical structure allows for nuanced expressions of profound spiritual concepts and for the capacity to communicate deep cultural and philosophical connections. The language's rich symbolism and metaphorical expressions convey intricate spiritual ideas, distinguishing it from English and other modern languages, which, though expressive, lack Sanskrit's vibrational potency.

Each component of every word in Sanskrit, when pronounced and intoned correctly, is said to activate different elements of our energy systems directly with specific vibrations. We know this because the lengthy spiritual texts that are the source for many mantras—such as the Vedas and Upanishads—were passed down with astonishing fidelity through an exacting oral tradition. Millennia spent with these special phrases revealed they could reliably encapsulate unique devotional moods, address specific ailments, and generate desired mind-states. Additionally, because they have been passed down through eons of human history, many well-known mantras carry a collective energetic imprint. And who wouldn't want to fill their being with vibratory medicine passed down through the ages?

Often, it seems, when we are not speaking a full truth, our options for speech feel narrow, jagged, and small. Remember a time in a job interview, public speaking, or on a first date when you felt the need to censor yourself and hold back your true feelings. This closing down of the throat chakra can become a lifelong pattern. By toning and even singing—through mantra—we can activate the physical pathways to break this pattern. The voice box opens. The muscles around the throat relax. The vocal cords warm and lengthen. When you add time-honored sacred phrases from any spiritual tradition, you multiply the mantra's healing potential and plant an energetic seed deep in your psyche. With regular chanting of sacred sounds, your voice will get stronger, and so will your confidence in your creativity and speaking your truth, thereby unlocking realms of possibility.

PRACTICE

START SIMPLY WITH THE ESSENCE

The meditative practice of chanting aloud can be extraordinarily pleasurable when the throat chakra is open and awake. The whole body becomes a vibrating speaker for sacred sound, affecting our own biochemistry and that of those around us. Sound good to you? Let's start small, with a single sound.

Every chakra has a "seed syllable" or bija mantra associated with it. As our awareness grows more subtle, it is said that many other seed syllables can be heard and utilized. The primary bija mantra for the throat chakra is *Ham*, pronounced "hum." When this sound is chanted repeatedly and with the awareness drawn to the physical throat area, it will activate your throat chakra.

Take a moment to sit at your altar or in some other quiet location where you will not be disturbed and where you will not feel self-conscious about your voice being heard by others. Take a few deep, clearing breaths, consciously releasing as much tension as possible from the body while keeping the spine straight. You want to feel that the chest and throat are physically open. No slouching!

Begin to warm up the vocal cords and diaphragm with the long, reverberant sounds of "ah" (pronounced as in the word *god*) on your exhalations. Find a note that is natural to you, not too high and not too low. Chant with the power of the belly and feel the sound reverberating in the chest cavity. Repeat ten times.

Now set a timer for five to ten minutes. Bring your awareness to the whole throat and neck area, from the collarbone to the jaw. If you can't quite feel this area, it can be helpful to place one or both hands over the throat or collarbone. Breathe in deeply and chant in the same way, using the sound of "hum" for the full length of the exhalation. Keep going and feel the vibration of this bija mantra in the throat and chest. Soften yourself while keeping a straight spine, and imagine feeling the sound all over your body. Is it possible to feel it in your feet?

Imagine the sound breaking up any tension and fear that are encasing the throat. Yes, I give you full permission to sing out and let go into this practice. Grow louder. Sound bolder. When your time ends, take a moment to notice how you feel and let it register in your experience.

Often, I find an external tone helpful in chanting because it engages my listening and helps me nestle into resonance rather than thinking about my pitch. In Western music, G is the musical note most often associated with the throat chakra. Use an instrument if you play one, or search on the internet for a video or sound file of this tone to chant with. Whatever you do, listen to the sound your voice creates. The ears are almost as important to the throat chakra as the voice, and when you engage both in balance, you will feel the magic.

PRACTICE

DEEPENING THE SEED

Now let's take this practice deeper to increase your awareness of your throat chakra. Perform the exercise just as before, and include the following guidelines.

First, when chanting *Ham*, focus on the "ah" sound for a few rounds. Open the mouth wide. Feel the vibration, specifically in the chest and torso. Smooth the rough and weak parts of the sound.

Next, close the lips and focus on the "mmm" of *Ham*, feeling vibrations in the hard palate of the mouth and in the sinuses. Keep the jaw relaxed, then bring your awareness to the "hhh" sound at the beginning of the bija mantra. Place some emphasis on it as if you were fogging the lenses of your glasses or laughing ("ha ha ha" or "ho ho ho").

Finally, put the three parts together. Engage the diaphragm with "hhh" while allowing the wide-mouthed "ahh" and the close-lipped "mmm" to advance in succession. Repeat and repeat.

Let this simple seed sound work through your entire vocal system. Close this practice as you did before by noticing how you feel. What has changed?

PRACTICE

WORK WITH A TRADITIONAL MANTRA

According to Hindu philosophy, there are three great forces in the universe: the creative (Brahma), the preservative (Vishnu), and the destructive (Shiva). Between the creation and the inevitable destruction before the next round of creation, there is a sustaining force that everything we can fathom depends upon for its continued existence.

For many Hindu Vaishnava traditions (those that worship the preserver deity Vishnu) the *mahamantra,* or "great mantra," is of unequivocal importance. Devotees know that chanting it with a sincere heart can lead to a closer connection with God and a state of spiritual bliss. The mantra is not only a means of seeking blessings but also a form of expressing love and surrendering to the Divine. In essence, the three Sanskrit names of God in this sixteen-word mantra point to different aspects of Lord Vishnu.

Hare can be interpreted in different ways but is typically seen as a name addressing Hari (another name for Vishnu) directly. The two deities Krishna and Rama, both incarnations of Vishnu in separate historic ages, are two of the most popular in Indian spirituality. I encourage you to learn more about these great beings; some of the most important epics in human literature have been written about them. A fun fact: in classic iconography, the skin of Vishnu and his incarnations is blue, the color associated with the throat chakra.

This mantra written in anglicized letters is the following:

> *Hare Krishna Hare Krishna*
> *Krishna Krishna Hare Hare*
> *Hare Rama Hare Rama*
> *Rama Rama Hare Hare*

Follow the steps as in the first practice, finding space and preparing. Then repeat the entirety of the first practice using the mahamantra. Sing it in a comfortable monotone voice with good rhythm. You can eventually give it a tune you find delightful to sing. Be creative. I often find clapping or slapping my legs in rhythm helpful. If you feel moved to jump up and down with your hands over your head, I'd say it's working! The great part about this mantra is that its popularity means there are thousands of recordings available using myriad melodies, so a quick internet search will turn up plenty of audio and video to sing along with. Of course, there is nothing quite like singing with others. Look for local kirtan groups. This mantra is usually in the repertoire.

After you've spent a number of sessions over a couple of weeks with the bija mantra and the mahamantra, take stock of how things are going in your everyday life. Are you making yourself clear when you speak? Are you saying what you really mean? Do you ask for (or demand) what you want from others? Are you honest with yourself and your loved ones?

SUMMARY

This chapter underscores the significance of chanting and singing mantras as a fundamental practice for healing and awakening the throat chakra. You do not need to know anything about these special phrases for them to work; simply commit to a regular chanting practice. You will notice changes compared to when your energy system previously became stuck or when you were unclear about how to best use your voice. Try taking these practices on your next lone walk in the woods, chanting to the rhythm of your feet. Go ahead and sing loudly in the personal sound booth of your car on the interstate. When chanting mantra becomes a regular reflex, you will sense its vital power.

Finally, remember that these sacred words emerging from your lips into the heavy reality of our time have been drawn through thousands of years by the grace of some sustaining force—truly mysterious and wild.

12

COLORS AND SHAPES

GINA NICOLE

There are many creative ways to bring about fifth chakra fitness, the goals of which are to achieve honest self-expression, strong communication with the Spirit and angels, and a healthy throat area. I find fifth chakra expansion by using shapes and specific colors, and I'll show you how to do that in this chapter.

MY FIFTH CHAKRA JOURNEY

It was through my own fifth chakra work that I learned my calling as a subtle energy medicine practitioner: to help others discover their voice, recognize their unique message, and fully embody that message.

My fifth chakra journey took the form of a health issue. For many years I suffered from an illness centered in my thyroid. After trying a range of ineffective treatments, I came upon one of Cyndi's books that pinpointed such problems as relating to the fifth chakra, and in that book I also learned that the fifth chakra activates at ages six and a half to eight and a half. Thinking back to my small self of that age, I vividly recalled being told not to talk so much, a message that landed in my throat chakra. Through additional profound explorations of my throat chakra, I unearthed layers of past silencing, negative beliefs, and energetic densities.

At the time I made this fifth chakra–thyroid connection, I was a practitioner of feng shui, which is the art of placing beneficial colors and shapes in the environment, and over time I used my knowledge of subtle colors and shapes to transmute the energy around my fifth chakra. Within six months of beginning this work, my disease had disappeared.

You don't need to be a master of the healing arts to embrace the concepts and protocols in this chapter. The only prerequisite is to tune in to your body and recognize any imbalances. Let the following insights inspire you to align your fifth chakra.

WORKING WITH SHAPES

To start, let's explore how shapes can be employed to stimulate the energy of the throat chakra in your daily life.

The most common representation of the throat chakra is a circle inside an inverted triangle, which is then nestled in a sixteen-petaled lotus flower. The symbology of this chakra relays the continual flow of energy from the higher to the lower chakras, supporting us in sharing our own essential higher truths. Focus on this symbol in your mind whenever you feel like you are lagging in energy. In addition to exploring this traditional symbolism, you can employ the following five shapes. I have found them incredibly potent for supporting the fifth chakra.

Hexagon

BENEFITS: This shape encourages clarity and balance, supporting the throat chakra in maintaining a harmonious flow of energy to bring about the speaking of truth and efficient communication.

VISUALLY: A hexagon is a six-pointed shape. It has six sides, six edges, and six vertices.

QUALITIES WHEN OVERUSED: Too bold in speech.

Ladder

BENEFITS: Symbolizes progress, growth, and ascension. The ladder serves as a metaphor for the journey toward higher understanding. It also represents the connection between the lower and higher chakras and the earthly and spiritual realms. Embodying upward movement, it mirrors the journey of self-expression and communication while supporting us toward clear articulation.

VISUALLY: Ladders are composed of horizontal lines that rise upward between two vertical poles. You can picture an endless ladder or any number of rungs.

QUALITIES WHEN OVERUSED: Rambling, talking in circles, speaking aimlessly.

Dodecahedron

BENEFITS: Encourages elevated forms of communication and self-expression. Represents universal communication from divinely sourced energy. Can shift negative words into positive. Represents universal communication from divinely sourced energy and connects us with higher realms.

VISUALLY: A three-dimensional shape with twelve pentagonal faces.

QUALITIES WHEN OVERUSED: Ungrounded conversations.

Metatron's Cube[14]

BENEFITS: Can help bring structure, universal order, truth, and stability to our conversations and words. Aids us in speaking from an optimal perspective. Believed to hold transformative and balancing properties that align and harmonize.

VISUALLY: A complex geometric pattern that is composed of multiple interconnected circles.

QUALITIES WHEN OVERUSED: Possibly kundalini energy rising too rapidly.

Merkaba or Star Tetrahedron

BENEFITS: Helps us communicate from a place of spiritual evolution and expanded awareness. "Mer" translates to light, "ka" signifies the spirit, and "ba" denotes the physical body. The image brings light and spirit into our words and expression. Meditating on or visualizing this shape may aid in activating higher levels of consciousness related to communication.

---

14 Metatron's cube and the merkaba are sacred geometry symbols that look similar. Metatron's cube is a two-dimensional pattern symbolizing universal creation and interconnectedness, while the merkaba is a three-dimensional star shape associated with personal spiritual evolution.

VISUALLY: A powerful shape, the merkaba is made of two intersecting tetrahedrons that spin in opposite directions to create a third-dimension energy field.

QUALITIES WHEN OVERUSED: Chatty dreams, emotional conversations.

Having discussed the significance of shapes, a question arises: How do we effectively utilize them? The options are boundless. Explore the realm of possibilities. Following are two approaches for incorporating shapes.

PRACTICE

ATTUNEMENT THROUGH ACTIVATED JEWELS

One of my favorite ways to activate the throat chakra with shapes is by wearing them around my neck. Adorning yourself with throat chakra symbols in the form of necklaces or pendants serves as a continual reminder to focus on open communication and authentic self-expression. These adorned jewels become not only a stylish accessory but also a tangible source of energetic support, harmonizing your throat chakra and empowering you to embrace your voice. As you put on a necklace or amulet, amplify your intentions by saying the following three times:

I adorn this necklace with grace
to activate my throat from my authentic space.

USE SHAPES IN YOUR HOME

Find the throat chakra area of your home by imagining a tic-tac-toe grid over the floor plan of your home, room, or personal space. Starting with the doorway or entry point, find the bottom right-hand corner of the space. This is the sector that connects to your throat chakra. With intention, place the shapes you are attracted to from the featured list, in the form of sculptures or pictures, in this area. They can be obvious or hidden. Then speak the following affirmation over the shape:

I am in alignment with my space and
activate the throat chakra with grace.

• • • • • •

While I personally enjoy the two methods I just shared, feel free to experiment with shapes in whatever ways resonate with you. Keep in mind that there are no strict guidelines or wrong approaches. Embrace the freedom to play with symbolism, and explore various combinations to discover what feels most effective for your unique experience.

WORKING WITH COLOR

An alternative approach to activating and harmonizing your fifth chakra involves the use of color. Each chakra traditionally corresponds to a specific color. The fifth chakra is commonly linked with blue, renowned for enhancing vocal expression, promoting self-expression, fostering a connection with Spirit, and supporting the fifth chakra's subtle energies.

Thinking creatively, we can also explore the entire color spectrum. Color embodies energy, and energy manifests as color. In my observations, the interconnectedness of our collective humanity has shown that every subtle energy particle exists universally, every color encompasses all others, and each chakra reflects the entirety of the chakra system.

I've identified five colors that are particularly beneficial for activating the fifth chakra. As you delve into each hue, pay attention to its diverse representations and meanings.

Blue

Various shades of blue can promote clear communication, self-expression, and authenticity, enhancing balance and harmony.

> **QUALITIES WHEN OVERUSED**: Disclosing what is private, misplaced trust, tense words.

AFFIRMATIONS: In shades of blue, my words imbue. Clarity unfolds as communication stays true.

Purple

Purple presents both calming and stimulating qualities. It is made by combining tranquil blue and energetic red, which aid in fostering intuitive conversations. Purple also enables the release of inhibitions and facilitates open, authentic communication, encouraging individuals to speak their truth with clarity. It infuses all conversations with spiritual insight.

QUALITIES WHEN OVERUSED: Fragile conversations, arrogance, speaking without thinking.

AFFIRMATIONS: In the throat chakra's gentle purple glow, my voice resonates; I am authentically in flow.

Coral

Coral carries a harmonious balance, representing the fusion of calmness, acceptance, and vitality. It also symbolizes creativity, warmth, and enthusiasm in communication. Focusing on coral helps create a balanced and supportive environment for the throat chakra, promoting clear communication and creative self-expression. It is a supportive color for community and group discussions.

> **QUALITIES WHEN OVERUSED**: Immature, flighty, or erratic conversations.
>
> **AFFIRMATIONS**: In coral's ray, my words convey; optimism brightens, and warmth lights the way.

Orange

Orange injects enthusiasm into conversations, fostering a dynamic and engaging exchange. Associated with creativity and innovation, orange stimulates inventive thinking, making it an ideal choice for expressing new ideas. Its friendly and approachable aura promotes a positive and welcoming atmosphere, facilitating open and relaxed communication. Orange ensures that messages stand out, contributing to a memorable and impactful communication experience.

> **QUALITIES WHEN OVERUSED**: Distractions, restless communication.
>
> **AFFIRMATIONS**: In orange's hue, my voice rings true; communication flows confident and anew.

Magenta

Considered a powerful color for communication in spiritual contexts, magenta balances emotional energies, evokes creativity, and connects us with higher consciousness. It captures attention while fostering a sense of emotional equilibrium, allowing for communication that goes beyond the mundane so as to tap into deeper, more spiritual dimensions.

QUALITIES WHEN OVERUSED: Overstimulated, agitated, controlling communication.

AFFIRMATIONS: With magenta's light, my words find grace as communication flows in a divinely connected space.

• • • • • •

Harnessing the power of color at the fifth chakra can illuminate both self-expression and spirit communication. Combined with the previous shape exercises, integrating color into our surroundings—encompassing our homes, decor, and clothing—serves as a potent means of activating and attuning the throat chakra. Following are two effective approaches to infuse color into your practice for enhanced throat chakra alignment.

PRACTICE

BLENDING COLOR WITH SOUND

The throat chakra, resonating with the essence of sound, invites a vibrant atmosphere. Tune in to your favorite melodies, nature sounds, or the soothing tones of wind chimes while incorporating one of the colors listed in this chapter into your surroundings. Use a pillow, an article of clothing, or anything to blend color and sound. This simple practice not only uplifts your space with sound but also enhances visual harmony, fostering a balanced and vibrant energy flow in sync with your throat chakra.

DESIGN FOR THE THROAT CHAKRA

Arrange your living or working space using one or more colors listed in this chapter, as well as items that incorporate throat chakra shapes. Consider using decor items like rugs, cushions, or wall art featuring these colors and shapes.

Incorporating throat chakra shapes and colors into your daily life and practices can lead you on a transformative journey of self-expression, balance, and support for all physical aspects of the throat area.

Find shapes and colors that resonate with you, bring them into your space through decor or clothing, and enjoy the creative process. Consider creating a personal space, like an altar, adorned with these symbols to reinforce your commitment to genuine communication. Infuse your daily practices, such as meditation, with these elements, approaching the journey with curiosity.

SUMMARY

Intentionally adding or featuring specific shapes or colors related to your throat chakra can foster clarity, authenticity, and a harmonious energy flow. Dive into these symbolic languages to unveil your throat chakra's potential for creativity and connection, contributing to a more vibrant and balanced life.

13

RECIPES

Welcome to the harmonious realm of the fifth chakra, the center of personal truth, nestled at the base of the throat. It's a genuinely mystical vortex where thoughts transform into words, where silence speaks volumes, and where the unspoken finds its voice. In this chapter, we dive into the foods of the fifth chakra, exploring their essence and culminating in a trio of plant-based recipes that can feed your fifth chakra and soul.

This chakra is associated with blue, symbolizing serenity, clarity, and creative expression. The ether element of the throat chakra emphasizes the importance of spaciousness and openness for clear communication. When the fifth chakra is in harmony, it empowers one to speak the truth confidently and listen with empathy and understanding, so blue-based foods are essential to supporting your communication skills.

THROAT-NOURISHING BLUE FOODS

Though there are not as many blue foods in the world to choose from as other colors, I *love* blue foods, especially blueberries, the superfood I devour on yogurt or gluten-free steel-cut oats many times a week. Further, I have a gastronomical fondness for roasted blue potatoes for lunch and dinner, and acai and butterfly pea flower powder in my morning smoothies. I also love the flavor and nutritional benefits of sea veggies such as wakame, nori, and arame.

Here is a partial list of some of the foods that balance the fifth chakra and are predominantly blue or blue-tinged:

» blueberries

» blackberries

» boysenberries

» purple grapes

» plums

» figs

» acai berries

» sea vegetables

» blue corn

» blue potatoes

» butterfly pea flower

» blue cauliflower

Blue foods are not just a feast for the eyes; they are a symphony of health benefits that perfectly align with the needs of the fifth chakra:

HARMONIZING THE THROAT AND THYROID: Blue foods are known for their soothing and healing properties, particularly beneficial for the throat and thyroid gland. This area of our body is crucial for communication and expression, and maintaining the health of this area is essential for the pure nectar chakra's balance.

FACILITATING FLUID COMMUNICATION: These foods nourish us physically and energetically and support clear, honest communication. By strengthening the throat area, they enable us to voice our thoughts and feelings more effectively, resonating with the essence of vishuddha.

CATALYSTS FOR CREATIVE EXPRESSION: Blue foods are believed to stimulate creativity, an essential aspect of the fifth chakra. They encourage us to express ourselves in unique and innovative ways, whether through speech, writing, art, or other forms of expression.

PACKED WITH NUTRITIONAL POWER: These foods are beautiful and dense in nutrients. They provide a range of vitamins, minerals, and other essential nutrients that support overall health and well-being.

RICH IN ANTIOXIDANTS: These foods' vibrant blue and purple hues come from their high antioxidant content, particularly anthocyanins. Antioxidants are crucial for combating free radicals, reducing inflammation, and supporting overall health.

BALANCING THYROID HORMONES: The thyroid gland, influenced by the fifth chakra, significantly regulates our energy and metabolism. Blue foods support thyroid function, helping maintain a balanced and energetic body.

Remember, flexibility and diversity are critical when deciding which foods to eat. Don't hesitate to expand your meal choices, try new foods and recipes, and be creative with your meals to maintain a healthy and vibrant throat chakra.

I recommend choosing organic food whenever possible and washing your fruits and vegetables to avoid unwanted dirt, debris, bugs, and pesticides.

To help diversify your home menu options and energize your heart chakra, here are three of my delectable, healthy, plant-based fourth chakra recipes: one each for breakfast, lunch, and dinner. Of course, you can mix and match and make these recipes at any time. Feel free to adapt them as your creativity and palate dictate.

Blueberry Bliss Breakfast Bowl

SERVES 1

This bowl of blue bliss will enhance your entire morning.

½ cup rolled oats (gluten-free optional)
1 tablespoon chia seeds
1 cup plant-based milk
1 cup fresh blueberries
1 banana, sliced
A drizzle of maple syrup
A sprinkle of cinnamon

Combine the oats, chia seeds, and plant-based milk in a bowl. Let the mixture sit overnight in the fridge. In the morning, stir the mixture and add more plant-based milk as needed. Top with blueberries, banana slices, maple syrup, and cinnamon.

Fantastic Fifth Chakra Power Bowl

SERVES 1

Boost your afternoon activities with energizing nutrition.

 1 cup cooked quinoa
 ½ cup shredded red cabbage
 ½ cup blueberries
 ½ cup blackberries
 1 small beet, roasted and sliced
 ½ avocado, sliced
 A handful of spinach or kale
 ¼ cup chopped walnuts
 2 tablespoons pumpkin seeds
 Your salad dressing of choice, homemade or store
   bought, to taste

Make your quinoa base by placing the cooked quinoa in a large bowl. Quinoa is a nutritious and versatile base, offering a subtle nutty flavor and a fluffy texture. Then begin to layer:

» Layer the shredded red cabbage over the quinoa. Its vibrant color and crunchy texture add both visual appeal and health benefits.

» Add the blueberries and blackberries. These berries are not just bursting with flavors but are also packed with antioxidants, aligning with the fifth chakra's energy.

» Place the roasted beet slices around the bowl. Beets bring a sweet, earthy flavor and a rich purple hue, enhancing the chakra theme.

» Gently lay the avocado slices on top. Avocado adds creaminess and is loaded with healthy fats, contributing to overall vocal health.

» Tuck in the spinach or kale leaves. These greens are nutrient powerhouses, adding a fresh, earthy component to the bowl.

» Sprinkle the chopped walnuts and pumpkin seeds over everything. These add a satisfying crunch and are rich in omega-3 fatty acids, which are great for brain health and, by extension, communication.

Drizzle the salad dressing over the power bowl. Then gently mix the ingredients in the bowl, or enjoy each component in its own right, exploring the unique flavors and textures.

SERVING SUGGESTION: Serve this fifth chakra power bowl with a glass of herbal tea, such as chamomile or peppermint, to further support throat health. Enjoy this meal in a peaceful setting, taking the time to savor each bite and reflect on the power of nourishment and mindful eating.

Vishuddha Harmony Stew

SERVES 1 TO 2

This hearty stew will prep you for evening ease and sleep.

- 1 tablespoon olive oil
- 1 medium onion, diced
- 2 cloves garlic, minced
- 1 cup cubed purple potatoes
- ½ cup sliced carrots
- ½ cup blue cauliflower florets (if available) or regular cauliflower
- ½ cup cubed eggplant
- ½ cup cooked black beans, drained
- 4 cups low-sodium vegetable broth
- 1 teaspoon dried thyme
- 1 teaspoon dried basil
- Salt and pepper to taste
- ½ cup coconut milk
- Fresh parsley for garnish
- Lemon wedges for serving

Sauté the base: Heat the olive oil in a large pot over medium heat. Add the diced onion and minced garlic, sautéing until they become translucent and fragrant. Stir in the potatoes and carrots and cook for about 5 minutes. Add the cauliflower and eggplant and continuing cooking for another 5 minutes.

Prepare the beans and broth. Mix in the black beans. Pour in the vegetable broth and bring the mixture to a low boil. Season with thyme, basil, salt, and pepper. These herbs not only add flavor but also support the throat chakra. Reduce the heat to a simmer and cook until the vegetables are tender, about 20 to 25 minutes.

Finish by stirring in the coconut milk for a creamy texture and a hint of sweetness, enhancing the stew's depth of flavor. Ladle the stew into bowls and garnish with fresh parsley. Serve with a wedge of lemon on the side, adding a refreshing and balanced citrus element.

SERVING SUGGESTION: Enjoy this vishuddha harmony stew with warm, crusty bread or a small serving of quinoa. The stew is hearty enough to be satisfying, but a grain accompaniment can add a comforting element.

PART 2: SUSAN WEIS-BOHLEN

Imagine a spectrum of blue shades sliding effortlessly down your throat. Included in this blue rainbow are various hues of nature's bounty that form a swirling mix in your mouth and then travel down your esophagus to your belly, where all those blue colors are happily and easily digested and assimilated into your blood, tissues, and organs. This sweet, pure nectar is further absorbed into your energy body, specifically your throat chakra.

Imbibing food that coats the throat with a warm, slippery elixir facilitates communication. This allows words, thoughts, and desires to flow from the mouth with greater ease. The recipes included here foster and support speaking your truth from the depths of the root chakra to the heights of the crown. The energies gather in the throat for the truest expression of your deepest desires. Eat, speak, and allow the bounty of your voice to be shared with the world.

There are more types of blue food than most people think. From blue corn to blue beans, purple/blue cabbage, and Tuscan kale, blue is all around us. These recipes might introduce you to some new foods. I've included dishes here that will delight with their simple preparation, robust nutrition, and chakra-balancing qualities.

Blueberry Spirulina Slippery Elm Elixir

SERVES 2

This drink will feel smooth and luxurious going down. Use warm liquid to enhance the throat coat. The slippery elm mixture is a pre- and probiotic mix that will please your belly. The combination is also helpful for calming acid reflux, which is a disturbance in the throat chakra when acid moves upward from the stomach to the esophagus to the throat. To keep the throat and voice clear and strong, it's ideal to calm excess acid.

½ cup slippery elm tea, warm:
  1 tablespoon slippery elm bark
  1 tablespoon marshmallow root
  1 teaspoon licorice root
1 cup fresh or frozen organic blueberries
1 teaspoon spirulina powder
1 cup warm oat or almond milk (can add more as needed)
1 small ripe banana
1 tablespoon coconut palm sugar or date sugar (optional)

Make the tea by grinding the herbs into a fine powder, or purchase them in powder form. Boil 3 cups of fresh, filtered water, add the powder, and mix well. Reduce and simmer until 2 cups of water are boiled off. Strain and use the thick, viscous liquid as a base for this smoothie or to sip on its own. These quantities will make a double batch. You can store the leftovers in an air-tight jar in the refrigerator for up to 3 days.

Add the tea and remaining ingredients to a blender and mix until smooth, about 30 seconds. Drink right away; the blueberries and slippery elm will become gelatinous if left to sit for a while. The mixture is also enjoyable as a pudding.

Smashed Blue Potatoes

SERVES 2

Blue potatoes, sometimes called purple potatoes, are packed with nutrients and contain acylated anthocyanins, a plant pigment that slows down the absorption of carbohydrates, leading to fewer spikes in blood sugar and reducing your chances of getting diabetes. Blue potatoes have a creamy, luscious texture that makes the mouth happy. When prepared this way, the outer blue skin crisps up, retaining the soft, smooth inside.

> 1½ pounds small to medium blue potatoes
> 3 tablespoons unsalted butter, melted
> 1 to 2 tablespoons avocado oil (or any high-heat oil)
> Flaky salt and black or white pepper to taste
> ½ cup fresh herbs to garnish before serving, such as scallions, cilantro, chives, parsley, rosemary or thyme, torn into pieces

Preheat the oven to 350°F. Wash the potatoes and boil them whole until soft, about 20 minutes. Drain and allow them to dry for about 15 minutes or until they are no longer steaming. Place them on an oiled baking sheet, with enough space between to allow them to cook fully, and smash them with a fork. Brush each one with some of the butter and oil, coating them well, and season with salt and pepper.

Place the baking sheet in the oven. Roast in the oven for about 40 to 45 minutes. Do not flip them. The skin should get crispy but not burn. Remove and immediately place on serving plates and top with the herbs. These are a super yummy treat on their own or as a side dish to any protein.

Blue Bean Salad with Roasted Blue Corn

Serves 2

Beans and corn are the superstars in this dish. Protein from Ayocote Morado blue beans and a mix of carbs and fat make it supremely satisfying and healthy. This is a full meal on its own or as a side with meat or tofu.

1 medium green pepper

1 tablespoon olive oil or avocado oil, divided

6 scallions

Salt and pepper to taste

Kernels from 4 ears blue corn (you can also use regular corn), boiled in water for about 1 minute

1 tablespoon butter

2 cups cooked Ayocote Morado beans (prepare according to package directions)

¼ cup lime juice

1 teaspoon red chili powder

¼ cup sour cream

1 teaspoon ground cumin

½ cup Greek feta cheese

1 bunch cilantro, stems removed

Cut the green pepper in half, remove the seeds, and chop into 1- or 2-inch pieces. Heat a large skillet over medium heat until hot (about 30 seconds), add 1 teaspoon oil, and toss in the peppers and the chopped scallions, coating them well and charring slightly. Remove the peppers and scallions and place them in a bowl. Add some salt and pepper and mix to combine.

Using the same hot skillet, add another teaspoon of oil and toss in the cooked corn kernels, allowing them to char for about 5 to 6 minutes. Add the butter and mix well. Pour the corn into the bowl with peppers and scallions. Add the cooked beans and stir to coat.

In a small bowl, mix together the lime juice, chili powder, sour cream, and a pinch of salt. Add a tablespoon of water if needed to help the ingredients combine. Pour this mixture over the green pepper, corn, and beans and stir well, careful not to make the beans mushy.

Add the cumin and more salt and pepper to taste. Pour the mixture into a serving bowl or a platter, and garnish with feta cheese and cilantro.

Drunken Codfish

SERVES 2

Codfish fresh from the deep blue sea with a bit of wine, garlic, and lemon engages the throat chakra with its smooth, silky texture and warming flavors. Served with smashed blue potatoes or blue bean salad with roasted blue corn, it makes for an energetically balancing meal.

2 6-ounce codfish fillets
1 tablespoon olive oil
1 large shallot or 2 small ones, thinly sliced
2 large garlic cloves, thinly sliced
½ cup water
8 ounces white wine
1 lemon, sliced

Heat a saucepan large enough for the two fillets over medium heat. When the pan is hot, add the oil and wait about 30 seconds for it to heat up but not smoke. Add sliced shallots and cook for about 3 minutes. Then add the garlic, thinly sliced, and stir for about 30 seconds, being careful not to let it burn. Add the water, wine, and lemon slices and stir. Allow the mixture to heat to a low boil, reduce the heat slightly, and then lay the cod in the pan and cover for about 5 minutes. Flip the cod and cook for another 5 minutes. At any time, you can check to test the consistency of the fish with a fork; when it flakes easily and is white through and through, it's done.

· · · · · ·

These pure nectar recipes will smooth and activate your throat chakra. Entice yourself into excellent communication with one of the most enjoyable activities in life: eating.

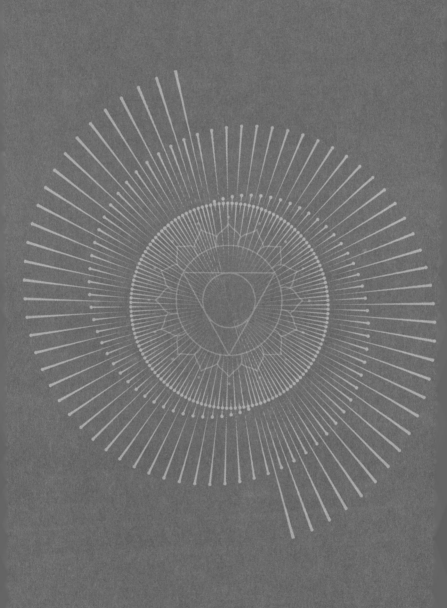

CONCLUSION

You started your expedition with a story about good and evil and the promise of purification via your fifth chakra. No matter what divine authority initially granted humankind the ability to transmute life's poisons, this book has treated you to antidotes for the woes of the world. Principles like honesty, soul, truth, and expression have been bringing you to the ultimate place of surrender: the acceptance of grace available through your throat chakra.

How satisfying to drink these energies from your own pure nectar chakra! Called vishuddha in Sanskrit, this swirling blue energy center is now busily helping you integrate its many gifts, foremost those of communication.

While enabling verbal exchanges, both psychic and conversational, your throat chakra also instructs you in good listening. It's not enough to hear another or simply bask in their silence. We must be capable of knowing what is really meant so we can respond to hidden meanings. A capable fifth chakra deepens this capacity for meaningful, accurate communication, and, therefore, loving connection. We can rest assured that this chakra, when healthy, is also creating health for its related bodily areas, including the throat, cervical vertebrae, and thyroid.

And as you've learned, you've only to imagine a brilliant blue energy, or to chant the bija *Ham,* to cleanse and renew it properly.

Throughout part 1 you were treated to the key points related to your throat chakra. You explored yantras and seed carriers, intuitive aptitudes and psychological assets, while lighting your soul from within. These touchstones prepared you for the next stage of the journey.

In part 2 you moved into personal growth. Imagine how empowered you now are, having acquired wisdom about—and participated in practices devoted to—fifth chakra spirit allies, yoga exercises, body awareness activities, meditations, vibrational remedies, sound techniques, cooking experiences, and so much more.

Ruminate for a little while longer, if you would, and think about how you might continue this pure nectar chakra adventure. What might you desire to further research, read, or experience? Your soul stands ready to assist you in making these choices, as does this book. After you've closed its pages, you can easily open them again.

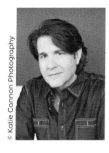

© Katie Cannon Photography

ANTHONY J. W. BENSON serves as a creative business strategist, manager, coach, producer, and writer specializing in working with consciously awake authors, speakers, musicians, entrepreneurs, and small and large businesses. He has shared his expertise on numerous podcasts and radio and television shows. Anthony has led a mindful plant-based lifestyle for over thirty-five years.

ANTHONYJWBENSON.COM
INJOICREATIVE.COM

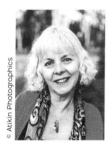

© Atikin Photographics

JO-ANNE BROWN is an intuitive, energy healer, and author who lives in central Queensland, Australia, with a background including engineering and bioresonance therapy. She helps highly sensitive people find meaning in their profound emotional experiences and release disharmonious patterns. She is featured in the internationally bestselling multi-author book *Intuitive: Speaking Her Truth*.

JOANNEINTUITIVE.COM

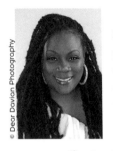

© Dear Davlon Photography

LINDSAY FAUNTLEROY is a licensed acupuncturist and founder of The Spirit Seed, a school that offers personal and professional development courses that are rooted in ancestral understandings of health, humanity, nature, and the cosmos. Lindsay is a certified instructor for the National Certification Commission for Acupuncture and Oriental Medicine (NCCAOM), as well as a facilitator of the Flower Essence Society's global practitioner certification program.

OCEANSANDDRIVERS.COM
THESPIRITSEED.ORG/INOURELEMENTBOOK

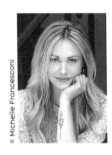

© Michelle Francesconi

AMANDA HUGGINS is an anxiety and mindfulness coach, certified yoga instructor, podcast host, author, and speaker. Her signature "Scientific, Spiritual, Practical" approach has helped thousands achieve transformation in mind, body, and soul. Besides presenting online courses, Amanda offers guidance on her podcast, *Anxiety Talks with Amanda*, and has an online community of over a half million followers.

INSTAGRAM AND TIKTOK @ITSAMANDAHUGGINS
AMANDAHUGGINSCOACHING.COM

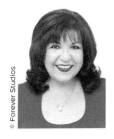

MARGARET ANN LEMBO is the author of *The Essential Guide to Crystals*, *Chakra Awakening*, *Animal Totems and the Gemstone Kingdom*, *The Essential Guide to Aromatherapy and Vibrational Healing*, *Angels and Gemstone Guardians Cards*, *Gemstone Guardians and Your Soul Purpose*, among other titles. She is an award-winning aromatherapist and the owner of The Crystal Garden, the conscious living store and center of the Palm Beaches.

MARGARETANNLEMBO.COM
THECRYSTALGARDEN.COM

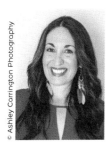

GINA NICOLE is a feng shui consultant, subtle energy medicine practitioner, and the author of a deck of wisdom cards. She encourages empathic people to orient their minds, bodies, spirits, and homes to align with higher frequencies to make impeccably clear and intuitive decisions. She loves to travel and is devoted to bringing transformational light to the foster care system.

GINANICOLE.NET

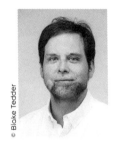

BLAKE TEDDER is a yoga instructor, musician, and guide who helps people connect to life and health by holding sacred spaces with movement, ritual, sound, and song. He hosts a podcast with yoga legends Angela Farmer and Victor van Kooten, a weekly radio show exploring contemplative musical landscapes, and, formerly, the internationally acclaimed *Full Lotus Kirtan Show*. He writes songs and leads chanting groups when not attending to his full-time work for a university research forest.

BLAKETEDDER.COM

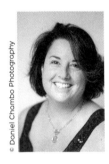

AMELIA VOGLER is an energy medicine and grounding specialist, internationally respected teacher of energy medicine, spiritual coach, and meditation guide. She embeds essential energetic practices in her meditations and teachings to better humanity. Maintaining an international private practice, she has helped thousands of individuals transform through grounding practices, intuitive insight, and advanced energy medicine.

AMELIAVOGLER.COM
VOGLERINSTITUTE.COM

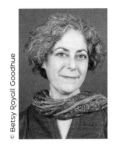

SUSAN WEIS-BOHLEN is certified in Ayurveda from the Chopra Center and has studied with Dr. Vasant Lad and Amadea Morningstar. She has also served on the National Ayurvedic Medical Association (NAMA) Board of Directors since 2018. A former bookstore owner, Susan is also the author of *Ayurveda Beginner's Guide: Essential Ayurvedic Principles and Practices to Balance and Heal Naturally* and *Seasonal Self-Care Rituals: Eat, Breathe, Move, and Sleep Better—According to Your Dosha*.

BREATHEAYURVEDA.COM

TO WRITE TO THE AUTHOR

If you wish to contact the author or would like more information about this book, please write to the author in care of Llewellyn Worldwide and we will forward your request. Both the author and the publisher appreciate hearing from you and learning of your enjoyment of this book and how it has helped you. Llewellyn Worldwide cannot guarantee that every letter written to the author can be answered, but all will be forwarded. Please write to:

Cyndi Dale
Llewellyn Worldwide
2143 Wooddale Drive
Woodbury, MN 55125-2989

Please enclose a self-addressed stamped envelope for reply or $1.00 to cover costs. If outside the USA, enclose an international postal reply coupon.

• • • • • •

Many of Llewellyn's authors have websites with additional information and resources. For more information, please visit our website:

WWW.LLEWELLYN.COM